The Medicalization of Society

The Medicalization of Society

*On the Transformation of Human Conditions
into Treatable Disorders*

PETER CONRAD

The Johns Hopkins University Press
Baltimore

2 4 6 8 9 7 5 3 1

The Johns Hopkins University Press
2715 North Charles Street
Baltimore, Maryland 21218-4363
www.press.jhu.edu

Library of Congress Cataloging-in-Publication Data

Conrad, Peter, 1945–
The medicalization of society : on the transformation of human
conditions into treatable disorders / Peter Conrad.
p. ; cm.
Includes bibliographical references and index.
ISBN-13: 978-0-8018-8584-6 (hardcover : alk. paper)
ISBN-10: 0-8018-8584-1 (hardcover : alk. paper)
ISBN-13: 978-0-8018-8585-3 (pbk. alk. paper)
ISBN-10: 0-8018-8585-X (pbk. alk. paper)
1. Social medicine—History.   I. Title.
[DNLM: 1. Sociology, Medical—trends. WA 31 C754m 2007]
RA418.C686 2007
362.1—dc22
2006033235

A catalog record for this book is available from the British Library.

For Irving Kenneth Zola (1935–1994) —
Pioneer in the study of medicalization,
inspiring colleague, and good friend

Contents

Preface

I have been interested in the medicalization of society for a long time. My Ph.D. dissertation was a participant observation study of the medicalization of hyperactivity in children (Conrad, 1976). This was followed by a more historical account of the medicalization of deviance, coauthored with Joseph Schneider (Conrad and Schneider, 1980). Then, after a decade studying other sociological issues, I again turned my attention to medicalization with a review article on medicalization and social control (Conrad, 1992). For nearly another decade, I didn't write much on medicalization, until I wrote a piece that fused my research on the public discourse of genetics with medicalization (Conrad, 2000).

Approaching the millennium, it was becoming clear to me that there were significant changes occurring around medicalization, and my interest, which had never waned, was piqued again. My intellectual focus had grown beyond deviance, so I knew I wanted to study the broader issues around medicalization. My first thought was to write a comprehensive account of medicalization, reviewing and integrating everything that had been written on the subject, a kind of medicalization magnum opus. Once I started delving into the literature, it was clear that this was too large a task. Simply too many human problems have been medicalized and too many scholars—historians, sociologists, anthropologists, physicians, feminists, bioethicists, and others—had examined pieces of it to fit in one book.

But I felt it was time for a new sociological examination of medicalization, and I settled on examining the key writings on the subject and focusing my analysis on a number of cases that reflected different aspects of medicalization. My goal would be not comprehensive but strategic with respect to the cases I would examine and the medicalization issues I would raise. I have always been most comfortable looking at problems inductively, from the case to the more general conceptual understanding. I would use these cases to develop a greater understanding about the changes in medicalization, especially as they have occurred in the past three-plus decades.

In general, I chose cases that interested me. There are certainly many important instances of medicalization that I could have examined—-obesity, reproduction, sleep problems, myriad addictions, the expansion of depression or post-traumatic stress disorder, just to name a few—but I selected cases that seemed to reflect on significant changes in medicalization. My approach was to study the cases one by one and to engage graduate students as collaborators in the process. This has been a most rewarding experience and has resulted in a number of coauthored publications, which I note in the acknowledgments. These cases allow me to examine certain facets of medicalization: extension of medicalization, expansion of existing categories, biomedical enhancement as medicalization, and the continuity of a classic case of demedicalization. I built on these cases, intertwining other examples, to develop some new conceptual understandings. These are seen most clearly in the final two chapters of this book and in a separate article (Conrad and Leiter, 2004).

So now, after more than thirty years as a student of medicalization, I am more convinced than ever that this is a subject of great sociological significance and an accelerating trend that has important implications for society. I hope that this book will shed new light the topic and encourage others to examine the issues further.

Chapter 1 describes the characteristics of medicalization, briefly reviewing the rise of medicalization and some ongoing controversies, outlining some of the changes in medicine in the past twenty years, and introducing the importance of the creation of markets for medicalization. The next four chapters examine specific cases of medicalization, each with a particular conceptual issue: extension of medicalization from one to both genders; diagnostic expansion of a specific malady to encompass more populations; biomedical enhancement as a form of medicalization; and the potential for remedicalization. The final three chapters analyze the measurement of medicalization, the shifting engines that drive this phenomenon, and some of the consequences of medicalization for medicine, patients, and society.

The second through fourth chapters examine both the creation of a demand for new medical products and the roles played by the pharmaceutical industry, physicians, consumers, and insurers in the emergence of medical markets and the medicalization of human problems. Until recently, women's problems were much more likely to be medicalized than men's. Chapter 2 examines three recent cases in which men have increasingly been seen as a market for medical products. As a result, andropause, baldness, and erectile dysfunction have been medicalized to different degrees. Chapter 3 examines the rise of adult attention-deficit/hyperactivity disorder to demonstrate how an extant medical category can expand to include an entirely new population of people (adults) for what was considered largely a disorder of children and adolescents. This type of diagnostic expansion has its roots in medical claims-makers, consumer demands, and the growing markets of the pharmaceutical industry. It is increasingly evident that the potential of biomedical enhancement will increase medicalization. Chapter 4 analyzes the case of human growth hormone, which has been at various times proposed as a medical enhancement for idiopathic short stature, aging, and athletic performance. Such biomedical enhancement is a particular form of medicalization that is likely to increase as science (especially genetics) develops new interventions to "improve" body and performance that are tempting to consumers and profitable for biotechnology companies. Chapter 5 first reviews the important example of the demedicalization of homosexuality and then evaluates the impact of several changes in medical knowledge, the gay and lesbian movement, and society that could lead to a remedicalization. While medical markets play a smaller role, biotechnology may still be a catalyst for remedicalization.

The next three chapters focus on issues that are more general to medicalization. Chapter 6 takes on the issue of measuring medicalization: how much medicalization is there, and how can we measure it? The growing number of medicalized categories indicates that medicalization is expanding, yet numbers are hard to locate. This chapter presents three ways to estimate increasing amounts of medicalization. Chapter 7 focuses on the emergent engines of medicalization. In the past thirty years, the driving forces behind medicalization have shifted from the medical profession, social movements, and inter- or intraorganizational conflicts to biotechnology, consumers, and managed care. In this chapter I focus on the importance of the creation of medical markets for medicalization. Chapter 8, the final chapter, analyzes some of the consequences of medicalization for our culture, society, medicine, and patients/consumers. In part in response to the spread of medicalization and its implications, pockets of resistance to medicalization have emerged, and these may be harbingers for the future.

Acknowledgments

I have researched and written about medicalization on and off for more than thirty years. In that time I have garnered many intellectual debts, far too many for me to remember and thank here. So here I will acknowledge and thank those many individuals who have aided the research, writing, and analysis of this book.

Earlier versions of several chapters first appeared as articles published in books or journals. Several of these were coauthored with some of the splendid students I have had the privilege to teach and work with at Brandeis University. Most of chapter 2 appeared first in a chapter coauthored with Julia Szymczak with part from another article written with Valerie Leiter; chapters 3 and 4 appeared first in slightly different form and were coauthored with Deborah Potter; chapter 5 was published in a shorter form coauthored with Alison Angell; a section of chapter 6 comes from collaborative work with colleagues Cindy Parks Thomas and Elizabeth Goodman and with Rosemary Casler; a small part of chapter 7 was coauthored with Valerie Leiter. Research done with Cheryl Stults and Heather Jacobson appears in chapter 6. I want to thank all of these students and colleagues for their contributions to this volume. I literally couldn't have done it without them. I hope they are pleased with how the work has been updated for the book.

I also want to thank Sharon Hogan, who was a great adviser and editor in helping me turn published journal articles into some of the core chapters of this book, and Elizabeth Ginsburg, for organizing and tracking down citations and references. I also thank Wendy Harris, my editor at Johns Hopkins University Press, for her support and patience while I was working to meet deadlines to complete the book. I am grateful to Mary V. Yates for her careful copy-editing.

A number of colleagues read chapters or excerpts at the manuscript stage and provided useful comments, which I most often heeded to the benefit of the book. These include Renee Anspach, Charles Bosk, Phil Brown, Michael Bury, Steve Epstein, Emily Kolker, Allan Horwitz, Susan Markens, Peter Nardi, Dana Rosenfeld, and Stefan Timmermans. I thank all these friends and colleagues and apologize in advance to anyone I inadvertently left out. None of these generous people is responsible for any shortcomings that remain.

Some of the material in this volume was previously published. I acknowledge the original publication outlets for permission to include the material here. Chapter 1 includes material that was published in the *Annual Review of Sociology*, *The Handbook of Medical Sociology* (Prentice Hall), and *Journal of Health and Social Behavior*; chapter 2 appeared in a different form in *Medicalized Masculinities* (Temple University Press) and *Journal of Health and Social Behavior*; chapters 3 and 4 appeared in a slightly different form in *Social Problems* and *Sociology of Health and Illness*; chapter 5 appeared in a much shorter and less fully developed form in *Society*; a section of chapter 6 is based on research we published in *Psychiatric Services*; an earlier version of chapter 7 appeared in *Journal of Health and Social Behavior*; and a few paragraphs in chapter 8 were published in *Annual Review of Sociology* and *The Handbook of Medical Sociology*. Thanks to all the publishers for allowing me to reprint and update the material here.

I want to acknowledge Brandeis University for a supportive academic environment, for several Mazer Faculty Grants, and for providing a sabbatical leave that greatly moved the project forward.

Finally, I thank my family for love and support, and especially my wife, Libby Bradshaw, who is at once a knowledgeable and sensible physician, a sounding board (and sometime critic) for my ideas, and a great life partner.

PART ONE

Concepts

CHAPTER ONE

Medicalization

Context, Characteristics, and Changes

When I began teaching medical sociology in the 1970s, the terrain of health and illness looked quite different from what we find in the early twenty-first century. In my classes, there was no mention of now-common maladies such as attention-deficit/hyperactivity disorder (ADHD), anorexia, chronic fatigue syndrome (CFS), post-traumatic stress disorder (PTSD), panic disorder, fetal alcohol syndrome, premenstrual syndrome (PMS), and sudden infant death syndrome (SIDS), to name some of the most prevalent. Neither obesity nor alcoholism was widely viewed in the medical profession as a disease. There was no mention of diseases like AIDS or contested illnesses like Gulf War syndrome or multiple chemical sensitivity disorder. While Ritalin was used with a relatively small number of children and tranquilizers were commonly prescribed for certain problems, human growth hormone (hGH), Viagra, and antidepressants like selective serotonin reuptake inhibitors (SSRIs) were not yet produced.

In the past thirty years or so, medical professionals have identified several problems that have become commonly known illnesses or disorders. In this book I address illnesses or "syndromes" that relate to behavior, a psychic state, or a bodily condition that now has a medical diagnosis and medical treatment. Clearly, the number of life problems that are defined as medical has increased enormously. Does this mean that there is a new epidemic of medical problems or that medicine is better able to identify and treat already existing problems? Or does it mean that a whole range of life's problems have now received medical diagnoses and are subject to medical treatment, despite dubious evidence of their medical nature?

I am not interested in adjudicating whether any particular problem is *really* a medical problem. That is far beyond the scope of my expertise and the boundaries of this book. I am interested in the social underpinnings of this expansion of medical jurisdiction and the social implications of this development. We can examine the medicalization of human problems and bracket the question of whether they are "real" medical problems. What constitutes a real medical problem may be largely in the eyes of the beholder or in the realm of those who have the authority to define a problem as medical. In this sense it is the viability of the designation rather than the validity of the diagnosis that is grist for the sociological mill.

The impact of medicine and medical concepts has expanded enormously in the past fifty years. To take just two common indicators, the percentage of our gross national product spent on health care has increased from 4.5 percent in 1950 to 16 percent in 2006, and the number of physicians has grown from 148 per 100,000 in 1970 to 281 per 100,000 in 2003 (Kaiser Family Foundation, 2005: Exhibit 5-7). The number of physicians per population nearly doubled in that period, greatly extending medical capacity. In this same period the jurisdiction of medicine has grown to include new problems that previously were not deemed to fall within the medical sphere.

"Medicalization" describes a process by which nonmedical problems become defined and treated as medical problems, usually in terms of illness and disorders. Some analysts have suggested that the growth of medical jurisdiction is "one of the most potent transformations of the last half of the twentieth century in the West" (Clarke et al., 2003: 161). For nearly four decades, sociologists, anthropologists, historians, bioethicists, physicians, and others have written about medicalization (Ballard and Elston, 2005). These analysts have focused on the specific instances of medicalization, examining the origins, range, and impact of medicalization on society, medicine, patients, and culture (Conrad, 1992; Bartholomew, 2000; Lock, 2001). While some have simply examined the development of medicalization, most have taken a somewhat critical or skeptical view of this social transformation.

In this chapter I examine some of the issues concerning medicalization and social control. Rather than summarizing the literature, I emphasize conceptual and substantive issues regarding medicalization. In doing so I make no attempt to provide a comprehensive review. Elsewhere I have reviewed some of the writings on medicalization more completely (Conrad, 1992, 2000).

CHARACTERISTICS OF MEDICALIZATION

Sociologists have studied medicalization since the late 1960s. The first studies focused on the medicalization of deviance (Pitts, 1968; Conrad, 1975), but soon the concept was seen to be applicable to a wide range of human problems that had entered medical jurisdiction (Freidson, 1970; Zola, 1972; Illich, 1976). To estimate the amount

TABLE 1.1
Searches on Medicalization, August 25, 2005

Google	71,700
Google Scholar	4,130 results
Social Sciences Citation Index	530 articles
Medline	445 articles
Social Science Abstracts	179 articles
Newspaper Abstracts	21 articles

of work that has been done on medicalization, I searched several databases with the keyword "medicalization." While the results of this search (see table 1.1) are only rough indices, they give a general sense of the amount of attention and writing given to this topic. In sociology alone there are dozens of case examples of medicalization; the corresponding body of literature has loosely been called the "medicalization thesis" (Ballard and Elston, 2005) or even "medicalization theory" (Williams and Calnan, 1996).

Medicalization also has gained attention beyond the social sciences. Numerous articles may be identified in a Medline search (of the medical literature), but of particular interest are the *British Medical Journal* (2002) special issue devoted to medicalization and an issue of *PLoS Medicine* (2006) largely devoted to "disease mongering." In 2003 the President's Council on Bioethics dedicated an entire session to examining medicalization (Kass et al., 2003). Less attention has been given to medicalization in the news, although the number of popular news references to medicalization has increased in the past couple of years. In 2005, for instance, the *Seattle Times* published a five-part investigative series entitled "Suddenly Sick" that focused on the promotion of illness categories and medicalization (Kelleher and Wilson, 2005). It seems evident that interest in and research on medicalization is growing as medicalization itself is increasing.

The key to medicalization is definition. That is, a problem is defined in medical terms, described using medical language, understood through the adoption of a medical framework, or "treated" with a medical intervention. While much writing, including my own, has been critical of medicalization, it is important to remember that medicalization describes a process. Thus, we can examine the medicalization of epilepsy, a disorder most people would agree is "really" medical, as well as we can examine the medicalization of alcoholism, ADHD, menopause, or erectile dysfunction. While "medicalize" literally means "to make medical," and the analytical emphasis has been on overmedicalization and its consequences, assumptions of overmedicalization are not a given in the perspective. The main point in considering medicalization is that an entity that is regarded as an illness or disease is not ipso facto a medical problem; rather, it needs to become defined as one. While the medical profession often has first call on most maladies that can be related to the body and to a large degree the psyche (Zola, 1972), some active agents are necessary for most problems to become medicalized (Conrad, 1992; Conrad and Schneider, 1992).

Many of the earliest studies assumed that physicians were the key to understanding medicalization. Illich (1976) used the catchy but misleading phrase "medical imperialism." It soon became clear, however, that medicalization was more complicated than the annexation of new problems by doctors and the medical profession. In cases like alcoholism, medicalization was primarily accomplished by a social movement (Alcoholics Anonymous), and physicians were actually late adopters of the view of alcoholism as a disease (Conrad and Schneider, 1992). And even to this day, the medical profession or individual doctors may be only marginally involved with the management of alcoholism, and actual medical treatments are not requisite for medicalization (Conrad, 1992; Appleton, 1995).

Although medicalization occurs primarily with deviance and "normal life events," it cuts a wide swath through our society and encompasses broad areas of human life. Among other categories, the medicalization of deviance includes alcoholism, mental disorders, opiate addictions, eating disorders, sexual and gender difference, sexual dysfunction, learning disabilities, and child and sexual abuse. It also has spawned numerous new categories, from ADHD to PMS to PTSD to CFS. Behaviors that were once defined as immoral, sinful, or criminal have been given medical meaning, moving them from badness to sickness. Certain common life processes have been medicalized as well, including anxiety and mood, menstruation, birth control, infertility, childbirth, menopause, aging, and death.

The growth of medicalized categories suggests an increase in medicalization (see chapter 6), but this growth is not simply a result of medical colonization or moral entrepreneurship. Arthur Barsky and Jonathan Boros point out that the public's tolerance of mild symptoms has decreased, spurring a "progressive medicalization of physical distress in which uncomfortable body states and isolated symptoms are reclassified as diseases" (1995: 1931). Social movements, patient organizations, and individual patients have also been important advocates for medicalization (Broom and Woodward, 1996). In recent years corporate entities like the pharmaceutical industry and potential patients as consumers have begun to play more significant roles in medicalization.

Medicalization need not be total; thus, we can say there are degrees of medicalization. Some cases of a condition may not be medicalized, competing definitions may exist, or remnants of a previous definition may cloud the picture. Some conditions such as death, childbirth, and severe mental illness are almost fully medicalized. Others, such as opiate addiction and menopause, are partly medicalized. Still others, such as sexual addiction and spouse abuse, are minimally medicalized. While we don't know specifically which factors affect the degrees of medicalization, it is likely that support of the medical profession, discovery of new etiologies, availability and profitability of treatments, coverage by medical insurance, and the presence of individuals or groups who promote or challenge medical definitions may all be significant in particular cases. There are also constraints on medicalization, including competing definitions, costs of medical care, absence of support in the medical profession, limits on insurance coverage, and the like. Medical categories can shift on the continuum toward or away from more complete medicalization.

Medical categories can also expand or contract. One dimension of the degree of medicalization is the elasticity of a medical category. "While some categories are narrow and circumspect, others can expand and incorporate a number of other problems" (Conrad, 1992: 221). For example, Alzheimer disease (AD) was once an obscure disorder, but with the removal of "age" as a criterion (P. Fox, 1989) there was no longer a distinction between AD and senile dementia. This change in definition to include cases of senile dementia in the population of adults over 60 years old sharply increased the number of cases of AD. As a result, AD has become one of the top five causes of death in the United States (cf. Bond, 1992). Medicalization by diagnostic expansion will be examined in chapter 3.

Medicalization is bidirectional, in the sense that there can be both medicalization and demedicalization, but the trend in the past century has been toward the expansion of medical jurisdiction. For demedicalization to occur, the problem must no longer be defined in medical terms, and medical treatments can no longer be deemed appropriate interventions. A classic example is masturbation, which in the nineteenth century was considered a disease and worthy of medical intervention (Engelhardt, 1974) but by the mid-twentieth century was no longer seen as requiring medical treatment. In a somewhat different vein, the disability movement has advocated, with partial success, for a demedicalization of disability and a reframing of it in terms of access and civil rights (Oliver, 1996). The most notable example is homosexuality, which was officially demedicalized in the 1970s; in chapter 5 I examine the possibilities of its remedicalization. Childbirth, by contrast, has been radically transformed in recent years with "natural childbirth," birthing rooms, nurse midwives, and a host of other changes, but it has not been demedicalized. Childbirth is still defined as a medical event, and medical professionals still attend it. Birthing at home with lay midwives approaches demedicalization, but it remains rare. In general, there are few contemporary cases of demedicalization to examine.

Critics have been concerned that medicalization transforms aspects of everyday life into pathologies, narrowing the range of what is considered acceptable. Medicalization also focuses the source of the problem in the individual rather than in the social environment; it calls for individual medical interventions rather than more collective or social solutions. Furthermore, by expanding medical jurisdiction, medicalization increases the amount of medical social control over human behavior. Early critics warned that medical social control would likely replace other forms of social control (Pitts, 1968; Zola, 1972), and while this has not occurred, it can be argued that medical social control has continued to expand. Although many definitions of medical social control have been offered, I still contend that "the greatest social control power comes from having the authority to define certain behaviors, persons and things" (Conrad and Schneider, 1992: 8). Thus, in general, the key issue remains definitional—the power to have a particular set of (medical) definitions realized in both spirit and practice. More recently critics have emphasized how medicalization has increased the profitability and markets of pharmaceutical and biotechnological firms (Moynihan and Cassels, 2005); these trends are discussed in later chapters. A fuller discussion of the social implications of the medicalization of society is found in chapter 8.

THE RISE OF MEDICALIZATION

Analysts have long pointed to social factors that have encouraged or abetted medicalization: the diminution of religion; an abiding faith in science, rationality, and progress; the increased prestige and power of the medical profession; the American penchant for individual and technological solutions to problems; and a general humanitarian trend in Western societies. These factors, rather than being explanatory, set the context in which medicalization occurs.

Most early sociological studies took a social constructionist tack in investigating the rise of medicalization. The focus was on the creation (or construction) of new medical categories with the subsequent expansion of medical jurisdiction. Concepts such as moral entrepreneurs, professional dominance, and claims-making were central to the analytical discourse. Studies of the medicalization of hyperactivity, child abuse, menopause, post-traumatic stress disorder, and alcoholism, among others, broadened our understanding of the range of medicalization and its attendant social processes (see Conrad, 1992). Michel Foucault (e.g., 1965), one of the great social analysts of the latter twentieth century, did not typically use the term "medicalization" but tended "to present a consonant vision that shows the impact of medical discourses on peoples lives" (Lupton, 1997: 94). But most studies of medicalization tend to be social constructionist rather than Foucauldian in orientation.

If one conducted a meta-analysis of the studies from the 1970s and 1980s, several social factors would predominate. At the risk of oversimplification, I suggest that three factors underlie most of those analyses. First, there was the power and authority of the medical profession, whether in terms of professional dominance, physician entrepreneurs, or, in its extremes, medical colonization. Here the cultural or professional influence of medical authority is critical. One way or another, the medical profession and the expansion of medical jurisdiction were prime movers for medicalization. This powerful medical authority was evident in the medicalization of hyperactivity, menopause, child abuse, and childbirth, among others. Second, medicalization sometimes occurred through the activities of social movements and interest groups. In these cases, organized efforts were made to champion a medical definition of a problem or to promote the veracity of a medical diagnosis. The classic example is alcoholism, with both Alcoholics Anonymous and the "alcoholism movement" central to medicalization of the condition (with physicians reluctant, resistant, or irresolute). Social movements were also critical in the medicalization of PTSD (W. Scott, 1990) and Alzheimer disease (P. Fox, 1989). Some efforts were less successful, as in the case of multiple chemical sensitivity disorder (Kroll-Smith and Floyd, 1997) and sexual addiction (J. Irvine, 1995). In general, organized grassroots efforts promoted medicalization. Third, directed organizational or inter- or intraprofessional activities promulgated medicalization, where professions competed for authority in defining and treating problems, as was the case with obstetricians and the demise of midwives (Wertz and Wertz, 1989) or the rise of behavioral pediatrics in the wake of medical control of childhood diseases (Pawluch, 1983; Halpern, 1990).

Far from medical imperialism, medicalization is a form of collective action. While physicians and the medical profession have historically been central to medicalization, doctors are not simply colonizing new problems or labeling feckless patients. Patients and other laypeople can be active collaborators in the medicalization of their problems or downright eager for medicalization (e.g., Becker and Nachtigall, 1992), although sympathetic professionals are usually needed for successful claims-making (Brown, 1995). Studies demonstrate the importance of the mobilization of people who are diagnosed in collectively promoting and shaping their diagnoses (e.g., Riessman, 1983). This kind of diagnostic advocacy is often accomplished in some association or connection with an extant social movement: PMS with the women's movement (Riessman, 1983; Figert, 1995); PTSD with the Vietnam veterans movement (W. Scott, 1990); and AIDS treatment with the gay and lesbian movement (Epstein, 1996). In each case the explicit politicization and mobilization of the social movement propelled the new category forward. Self-help and patient advocacy groups are legion, and some have promoted the acceptance of their own illness categories (Rossol, 2001; Barker, 2002).

To be sure, other contributing factors were implicated in the analyses. Pharmaceutical innovations and the marketing of Ritalin and hormone replacement therapy

(HRT) played a role in the medicalization of hyperactivity and menopause. Third-party payers (i.e., the health insurers that would pay for treatment) were factors in the medicalization of "gender dysphoria," obesity, and the detoxification and medical treatment for alcoholism. However, it is significant that in virtually all studies where they were considered, the corporate players in medicalization were deemed secondary to professionals, patient movements, or other claims-makers. By and large, the pharmaceutical and insurance industries were not central to the analyses.

Medicalization studies by sociologists and feminist scholars have shown how women's problems have been disproportionately medicalized. This is manifested in studies of reproduction and birth control, childbirth, infertility, premenstrual syndrome, fetal alcohol syndrome, eating disorders, sexuality, menopause, cosmetic surgery, anxiety, and depression. Catherine Kohler Riessman (1983) and Elianne Riska (2003) incisively examined the particular gendered aspects of medicalization. While the medicalization of women's bodies and difficulties continues (Lock, 2004), as discussed in chapter 2, men, especially aging male bodies, are now also being increasingly medicalized. While medicalization is not yet gender equal, it seems to be moving in that direction (e.g., Rosenfeld and Faircloth, 2006).

CONTROVERSIES AND CRITIQUES

Studies of medicalization have not been without controversy.[1] These controversies are important to moving the study of medicalization forward. But readers not interested in what may seem to be internal academic debates can skip this section and move to the next one. For those who stay the course there is the promise of a greater understanding of the contours of the medicalization process.

The earliest critiques argued that the medicalization case has been overstated and that significant constraints limit rampant medicalization (R. Fox, 1977; Strong, 1979). Some of these critiques conflated deprofessionalization with demedicalization (R. Fox, 1977). Others failed to recognize that most studies of medicalization adopt a historical, social-constructionist perspective. This perspective focuses on the emergence of medical categories and how problems entered the medical domain, bracketing whether a phenomenon is "really" a medical problem (Bury, 1986; see Conrad, 1992: 212). From a sociological perspective, case studies of medicalization have created a new understanding of the social process involved in the cultural production of medical categories or knowledge; however, these investigations do not necessarily contain a mandate as to how the categories and knowledge are to be evaluated.

In the 1990s several writers suggested ways of "rethinking" or "reconsidering" medicalization. For example, some noted how changes in society and medicine may place new constraints on medicalization. Simon Williams and Michael Calnan (1996) contended that most studies of medicalization viewed individuals or the lay public as largely passive or uncritical of medicine's expansion. They suggested that a better-informed public would create a "challenge of the articulate consumer." Barsky and Boros (1995) noted that despite a growing medicalization of bodily distress (e.g., somatization), managed care creates great incentives to reduce utilization, therefore placing new constraints on medicalization. While it remains questionable whether most studies of medicalization see the public as passive ("medical dupes," as Vicente Navarro [1976] put it many years ago), it seems clear that culture and medicine may limit medicalization. But as I endeavor to demonstrate in this book, perhaps especially in chapter 7, both articulate consumers and managed care incentives may promote as well as constrain medicalization. It is important to recognize that problems can still be medicalized, even in the face of skeptical members of the public or a medical system that resists treating them. For example, the fact that insurance companies won't pay for treatment of certain medical diagnoses limits medicalization but doesn't necessarily undermine it, so long as medical categories are accepted and applied to problems. It may, however, affect the degree of medicalization. Much of what is called self-care involves the use of medical approaches by lay people in the absence of professional medical treatment.

Most analysts of medicalization have written in a critical mode, either emphasizing the problems of overmedicalization or its consequences. Using the case of chronic fatigue syndrome, Dorothy H. Broom and Roslyn V. Woodward (1996) maintained that some writers have emphasized the downsides of medicalization and that medicalization can be both helpful and unhelpful to patients. They suggested, in the case of CFS, that medical explanations can provide coherence to patients' symptoms, validation and legitimation of their troubles, and support for self-management of their problems. Broom and Woodward distinguished medicalization from medical dominance (which they see as problematic for patients), and they called for a collaborative approach between the physician and the patient. They suggested that "constructive medicalization" is capable of improving the individual's well-being. In a sense, they echoed Catherine Kohler Riessman's (1983) point that medicalization can be a "two-edged sword" and my own depiction of the brighter and darker sides of medicalization (Conrad, 1975)—but they gave more credence to the benefits. It seems likely that certain benefits of medicalization will be more apparent with controversial illnesses like CFS, although as Talcott Parsons (1951) pointed out in his classic formulation of the sick role, medical diagnosis can legitimate a range of human troubles. Broom and Woodward (1996) departed from Parsons by suggesting that legitimation can occur with collaboration rather than through professional dominance. That is, physicians concurred with a patient's appeal for a medical diagnosis, rather than simply labeling a patients' condition as an illness.

Holistic health approaches are typically deemed alternative medicine and often are taken as a step toward demedicalization. After all, holistic approaches move away from the traditional medical model and frequently bypass the medical profession. June Lowenberg and Fred Davis (1994), using a broad conceptualization of medicalization, found that adaptation of holistic health does not by itself constitute evidence for either demedicalization or medicalization. Some aspects support medicalization (e.g., broadening the pathological sphere, maintaining a reshaped medical model), while others support demedicalization (e.g., reduction of technology and of status difference between providers and clients). Holistic health is frequently a form of deprofessionalization without demedicalization. Lowenberg and Davis found no unilateral movement in the direction of medicalization either way and rightly cautioned against simple generalizations. In recent years there has been a repositioning of complementary and alternative medicine (CAM) toward conventional medicine under the banner of "integrative medicine." This shift toward professionalization can been seen with the development of the National Center for Complementary and Alternative Medicine at the National Institutes of Health (www.nccam.nih.gov) and suggests a shift of alternative medicine in the direction of medicalization.

Simon Williams (2002, 2005) proposed that sleep provides another chapter in what he calls the medicalization-healthicization debate. By this he means that a variety of sleep disorders appear to have been subject both to medicalization and to healthicization (a rather awful word I coined a number of years ago [1992]) in terms of deeming the quantity and quality of sleep necessary for good health. Others (Hislop and Arber, 2003) claim, based on a small study of women, that sleep has been somewhat demedicalized as women use more "personalized strategies," perhaps akin to holistic health, in managing their sleep problems. But similar to Lowenberg and Davis's notion, personal or holistic solutions don't necessarily indicate demedicalization. I tend to align with Williams, at least in terms of the increasing medicalization of sleep, insomnia, and narcolepsy. These states have long been at least partly in the province of medicine, but now a whole array of sleep disorders (e.g., sleep apnea, shift work sleep disorder, sleep paralysis) have been identified. Recently there have even been advertisements in medical journals for the medication Provigal (modafinil) for "excessive sleepiness," for people who sometimes can't keep their eyes open during the day (cf. Wolpe, 2002; Kroll-Smith, 2003). My observation is that if this is a "disorder," it has a reasonably high prevalence among college students attending early or late classes!

Elsewhere, Williams contended that the more recent Foucauldian and post-modern critique has supplemented the standard socially constructionist-based medicalization conceptions. Williams contends, "Thus a new more thoroughgoing 'medicalization critique' has, in effect, emerged, in which the former acknowledgement or acceptance of an underlying 'natural' or 'biophysical' has itself been critically questioned or stripped away, if not abandoned altogether" (2001: 147).

Following Lupton (1997) and to a lesser degree Armstrong (1995), Williams acknowledges that both approaches focus on medicine as a dominant institution that has expanded its gaze and jurisdiction substantially in the past half-century or more. The Foucauldian view emphasizes more how the discourses of medicine and health become central to the subjectivities of people's lives, manifested as "the wholesale incorporation of the body and disease . . . in the discursive matter via the productive effects of power/knowledge, viewed as socially constructed entities" (Williams, 2001: 148). Without getting into a debate about the differences between a Foucauldian perspective and that presented in most medicalization studies, let me at least note some complementary lines of analysis. Medicalization studies, as I and others engage in them, focus especially on the creation, promotion, and application of medical categories (and treatments or solutions) to human problems and events; while we are certainly interested in the social control aspects of medicalization, we see them as something that goes beyond, but may include, discourse and subjectivity. Numerous studies have emphasized how medicalization has transformed the normal into the pathological and how medical ideologies, interventions, and therapies have reset and controlled the borders of acceptable behavior, bodies, and states of being. The medical gaze, discourse, and surveillance are fundamental elements of this process, even if these writers use a different vocabulary. It is clear that the postmodern critique points to the limits of modernist categorization, but it is the very processes of medical categorization that create medicalization. It is not necessary to adopt postmodern premises to be critical of the categorization of wide swatches of life into medical diagnoses or to adopt some relativist critique of medical viewpoints and cultural power. Foucault wrote about medicalization in one of his earlier works, *Birth of the Clinic:* "The two dreams (i.e., nationalized medical profession and disappearance of disease) are isomorphic; the first expressing in a very positive way the strict, militant, dogmatic medicalization of society, by way of a quasi-religious conversion and the establishment of a therapeutic clergy; the second expressing the same medicalization, but in a triumphant, negative way, that is to say, the volitization of disease in a corrected, organized, and ceaselessly supervised environment, in which medicine itself would finally disappear, together with its object and *raison d'être*" (1966: 32).

The medicalization thesis, as it is now constituted, focuses to some degree on both of these dimensions: it examines how medicine and the emerging engines of medicalization develop and apply medical categories, and to a lesser degree it focuses on how the populace has internalized medical and therapeutic perspectives as a taken-for-granted subjectivity (cf. Furedi, 2006). Indeed, most medicalization analysts contend that increasing parts of life have become medicalized and that medical or quasi-medical remedies are often explicitly sought for an expanding range of human difficulties. To put it crudely, medicalization of all sorts of life problems is now a common part of our professional, consumer, and market culture.

Adele Clarke and colleagues (2003), in an ambitious paper, endeavor to reconceptualize medicalization as "biomedicalization." By biomedicalization they mean "the increasingly complex, multisited, multidirectional processes of medicalization that today are being reconstituted through the emergent social forms and practices of a highly and increasingly technoscientific biomedicine" (Clarke et al., 2003: 162). These authors claim that this broader conceptualization of biomedicalization better captures the transformation of the organization and practices of Western biomedicine (see also Clarke et al., 2006). Their argument has many virtues, including alerting readers to changes affecting medicalization and the mounting structural and knowledge complexities of biomedicine. As should be apparent in this book, I agree with much of what Clarke and colleagues see as happening in medicine, but I believe it is better captured by acknowledging the shifting engines of medicalization (Conrad, 2005) and the increasingly market-based forms of medicalization (Conrad and Leiter, 2004). Biomedicalization is a much broader concept than medicalization and emphasizes a more extensive set of changes than is usually meant by medicalization, thus in my view compromising the focus on medicalization itself. Yet it seems clear that significant changes in medicine have had a significant impact on medicalization.

CHANGES IN MEDICINE

By the 1980s some profound changes in the organization of medicine were having important consequences for health matters. I can touch on them only briefly here. Medical authority eroded (Starr, 1982), health policy shifted from concerns of access to cost control, and managed care became central. As Donald Light (1993) pointed out, countervailing powers among buyers, providers, and payers changed the balance of influence among professions and other social institutions. Managed care, attempts at cost controls, and corporatized medicine changed the organization of medical care. The "golden age of doctoring" (McKinlay and Marceau, 2002) ended, and an increasingly buyer-driven system was emerging. Physicians certainly maintained some aspects of their dominance and sovereignty, but other players were becoming important as well. Large numbers of patients began to act more like consumers, both in choosing health insurance policies and in seeking out medical services (Inlander, 1998). Managed care organizations, the pharmaceutical industry, and some kinds of physicians (e.g., cosmetic surgeons) increasingly viewed patients as consumers or potential markets.

In addition to these organizational changes, new or developed arenas of medical knowledge were becoming dominant. The long-influential pharmaceutical companies comprise America's most profitable industry, and revolutionary new drugs expanded their influence (Angell, 2003; *Public Citizen*, 2003). By the 1990s the Human Genome project, the $3 billion venture to map the entire human genome, had been launched, with a draft completed in 2000. Genetics has become a cutting edge of medical knowledge and has moved to the center of medical and public discourse about illness and health (Conrad, 1999). The biotechnology industry has had starts and stops, but it promises a genomic, pharmaceutical, and technological future that may revolutionize health care (see Fukuyama, 2002).

Some of these changes have already been manifested in medicine, perhaps most clearly in psychiatry, where advances in knowledge have shifted the focus in three decades from psychotherapy and family interaction to psychopharmacology, neuroscience, and genomics. This shift is reinforced when third-party payers will pay for drug treatments but severely limit individual and group therapies. The choice available to many doctors and patient-consumers is not whether to have talking or pharmaceutical therapy, but rather which brand of drug should be prescribed.

Thus, by the 1990s enormous changes in the organization of health care, medical knowledge, and marketing had created a different world of medicine. How have these changes affected medicalization?

Adele Clarke and colleagues (2003) argue that medicalization is intensifying and being transformed. They suggest that around 1985, "dramatic changes in both the organization and practices of contemporary biomedicine, implemented largely through the integration of technoscientific innovations" (p. 161), coalesced in that expanded phenomena they call biomedicalization. Clarke and colleagues paint with a broad brush and in my view lose some of the focus on medicalization (see Conrad, 2005). But I agree there have been major changes in medicalization in the past two decades, and it is the purpose of this book to explore some of these shifts in medicalization and assess their consequences.

Many of the key studies of medicalization were completed over a decade or even two decades ago. This book examines some changes in medicalization that have occurred in the context of such important changes in medicine as the widespread corporatization of health care, the rise of managed care, the increasing importance of the biotechnological industry (especially the pharmaceutical and genomics industries), and the growing influence of consumers and consumer organizations. Some of these changes we see exemplified in expanding medical markets.

ON MEDICAL MARKETS

Sociologists have rarely looked at the growth of health care, much less the expansion of medicalization, in terms of markets. But when medical products, services, or treatments are promoted to consumers to improve their health, appearance, or well-being, we see the development of medical markets (see Conrad and Leiter, 2004). This should not be surprising, given our increasingly corporatized health system and the growing consumer culture for health-related products and services.

The use of advertising, the development of specific medical markets, and the standardization of medical services into product lines have contributed to an increased commodification of medical goods and services. Advertising of health care has become more commonplace (Dyer, 1997), and new medical markets have emerged, particularly for specialty services. Imershein and Estes (1996) argue that medical services are increasingly organized into product lines (with attached payment schemes), consistent with a market-based approach to exchange. Cosmetic surgery is the most commodified of medical specialties; it offers treatments such as liposuction and breast augmentation that are often not covered by insurance (Sullivan, 2001). Cosmetic surgeons advertise to stimulate demand for their services, for which patients pay either out of their own pockets or by borrowing from finance companies that partner with cosmetic surgeons, much as if they were purchasing a car.

In the last decade, a loosened regulatory environment has given pharmaceutical and biotechnology companies more freedom in advertising their wares, both to physicians and consumers. The Food and Drug Administration Modernization Act of 1997 (FDAMA) made several changes that have facilitated medicalization. Most relevant to our analysis, the act loosened the restrictions placed on the kind of information that pharmaceutical companies could share with physicians regarding "off-label" uses of their drugs. Subsequently, the amount of information that must be included in direct-to-consumer (DTC) advertisements has decreased. When the Food and Drug Administration (FDA) approves a drug, it can only be advertised for the specific disease and age group (e.g., adults) for which it has been tested. However, physicians may use any medications for any disorders or patients for whom they deem them appropriate; when it is not an FDA-approved indication, it is called an off-label use. FDAMA allowed pharmaceutical companies and their sales representatives to give physicians information about off-label uses so long as they provided adequate scientific documentation or were engaged in clinical trials for the new uses. Thus, the new regulations allowed the pharmaceutical companies to promote medications for off-label uses.

DTC advertising has increased since the 1980s, but the FDA requirement to list all potential risks and side effects limited such promotion to advertising in popular magazines, and even there with a great deal of small print describing effects. The risk requirement made it virtually impossible to do DTC advertising in broadcast venues. The 1997 regulation eased up on the requirement to include complete risk information. Advertisers were allowed to replace a long written list of risks with some manner in which the consumer could access the information (e.g., a website, a toll-free number, a print magazine ad). This change made DTC advertising on television possible, to the point that by 2004, $4.5 billion was spent per year advertising medications and focusing on the ills they are meant to treat (Conrad and Leiter, 2005; Hensley, 2005).

The constant development of new technologies, treatments, and drugs sparks consumer interest in obtaining access to these new medical goods and services, and advertising can further increase consumer demand. The pharmaceutical industry is becoming more directly involved in medicalization by using DTC advertising to create markets for its products; in doing so, it is medicalizing more aspects of life. The case of Paxil and social anxiety disorder provides a powerful illustration about how marketing directly to consumers has become part of the medicalization process.

The FDA approved Paxil (paroxetine hydrochloride) for the treatment of depression in 1996. Paxil followed Prozac and several other selective serotonin reuptake inhibitors (SSRIs) into an already saturated market for the treatment of depression. The manufacturer of Paxil (now called GlaxoSmithKline) responded to the saturated "depression market" by requesting FDA approval for additional applications of Paxil. The manufacturer chose to specialize instead in the "anxiety market," including panic disorder and obsessive compulsive disorder at first, and then social anxiety disorder (SAD) and generalized anxiety disorder (GAD). Paxil's application to SAD and GAD has contributed to the medicalization of emotions such as worry and shyness. While drug marketing is not the sole factor in the medicalization of shyness (S. Scott, 2006), it is a key example of how pharmaceutical marketing can reframe and medicalize common human characteristics and experiences.

SAD and GAD were fairly obscure diagnoses when they were added to the third edition of the American Psychiatric Association's *Diagnostic and Statistical Manual* (DSM-III) in 1980. According to the DSM-IV, SAD (or "social phobia") is a persistent and extreme "fear of social and performance situations in which embarrassment may occur" (APA, 1994: 411), and GAD involves chronic, excessive anxiety and worry (lasting at least six months), involving multiple symptoms (pp. 435–36). Both conditions are defined as being associated with significant distress and impairment in functioning. Horwitz (2002) notes how small changes in the wording of criteria for SAD resulted in a tremendous growth in its estimated prevalence (and potential market).

Marketing diseases and then selling drugs to treat those diseases is now common in the "post-Prozac" era. Since the FDA approved the use of Paxil for SAD in 1999 and for GAD in 2001, GlaxoSmithKline has spent millions of dollars on well-choreographed disease awareness campaigns to raise the public visibility of SAD and GAD. The pharmaceutical company's savvy approach to publicizing SAD and GAD, which relied upon a mixture of "expert" and patient voices, simultaneously gave the conditions diagnostic validity and created the perception that they could happen to anyone (Koerner, 2002). Soon after the FDA approved the use of Paxil for SAD, Cohn and Wolfe (a public relations firm that was working for what was then SmithKline) began putting up posters at bus stops with the slogan, "Imagine Being Allergic to People." Later in 1999 a series of ads featured "Paxil's efficacy in helping SAD sufferers brave dinner parties and public speaking" (Koerner, 2002: 61). Barry Brand, Paxil's product director, said, "Every marketer's dream is to find an unidentified or unknown market and develop it. That's what we were able to do with social anxiety disorder" (Vedantam, 2001).

Through media campaigns, GlaxoSmithKline redefined SAD and GAD, paradoxically, as both common (reducing the stigma associated with having a "mental illness") and abnormal (subject to medical intervention, in the form of Paxil). Prevalence estimates of both SAD and GAD range widely. For example, estimates of the prevalence of SAD range from 3 percent to 13 percent of the U.S. population (APA, 1994: 414), and the National Institute of Mental Health estimates that 3.7 percent of the U.S. population has SAD (Vedantam, 2001). Higher prevalence rates are associated with less stringent application of the DSM-specified criteria for these conditions.[2] Horwitz argues that "because community studies consider *all* symptoms, whether internal or not, expectable or not, deviant or not, as signs of disorder, they inevitably overestimate the prevalence of mental disorder in the community" (2002: 105). Likewise, the disease awareness campaign focused on individuals' feelings in social situations such as public speaking that were likely to evoke fear in many people, and it offered consumers symptom-based "self-tests" to assess the likelihood that they had SAD and GAD. This kind of clinical ambiguity is fertile ground for creating an expansive medical market.

Some question the validity of SAD because of its loosely defined boundaries and the aggressive marketing of it as a disease: "The impression often conveyed by commercials for the drugs is clear: almost anyone could benefit from them" (Goode,

2002: 21). Paxil's web page (www.paxil.com) stresses the elimination of symptoms (e.g., improved sleep) and improved performance (e.g., "improved ability to concentrate and make decisions") as benefits. Murray Stein, a psychiatry professor at the University of California at San Diego, has called the use of prescription medicines such as Paxil, which are costly and may have significant side effects, "cosmetic psychopharmacology" (Vedantam, 2001: 1).

Efforts to define SAD and GAD as conditions and market Paxil as a treatment for them have been extremely successful. Paxil is one of the three most widely recognized prescription drugs, after Viagra and Claritin (Marino, 2002), and in 2001 it was ranked ninth in terms of prescriptions (IMS Health, 2001), with U.S. sales of approximately $2.1 billion and global sales of $2.7 billion. Paxil sales declined somewhat after the patent expired in 2003 and cheaper generic versions became available. (It is, of course, not possible to distinguish how many of these prescriptions were for SAD or GAD and how many for other problems including depression, obsessive compulsive disorder, and post-traumatic stress disorder.)

But there has been a recent backlash against the drug. In 2002 a federal judge ordered a temporary halt to Paxil ads over the claim that Paxil is not habit forming (White, 2002). Apparently patients and health care providers have submitted thousands of reports to the FDA describing withdrawal symptoms (Peterson, 2002). Multiple lawsuits have been filed, asserting that physicians and consumers were misled by advertisements regarding the severity of withdrawal (Barry, 2002). In recent years there has been considerable public concern that Paxil may actually increase the risk of suicide among adolescents (Mahler, 2004), and along with several other SSRIs, it has been banned in the United Kingdom for use with children and adolescents. Like similarly marketed consumer goods such as trendy music and clothing, it is possible that Paxil's popularity may be waning. However, along the way, the GlaxoSmithKline campaign for Paxil has increased the medicalization of anxiety by implying directly and indirectly that shyness and worry may be medical problems and that Paxil is the way to treat them.

The case of Paxil demonstrates how pharmaceutical companies are now marketing diseases, not just drugs. This change is in part a result of the 1997 changes in FDA regulations that allowed for "educational" broadcast advertising that focuses on the disease or disorder, rather than on a specific drug, and in part as a result of the pharmaceutical industry's attempt to develop markets for its products. While physicians are still significant for medicalization—as reflected in the typical refrain, "Ask your doctor if [name of drug] is right for you"—we will see in subsequent cases that physicians' role in medicalization is decreasing as that of the pharmaceutical promoters is increasing.

PART TWO

Cases

CHAPTER TWO

Extension

Men and the Medicalization of Andropause, Baldness, and Erectile Dysfunction

Medicalization is dynamic and frequently can expand in new directions. One visible area of expansion is how aging men's lives and bodies are increasingly coming under medical jurisdiction. Television programs about successful aging, magazine articles about the best therapy for hair loss, and images used to promote the latest erectile dysfunction medication consistently tell men to "see your doctor." This movement of aging from a natural life event to a medical problem in need of treatment (Estes and Binney, 1989; S. Kaufman et al., 2004) is an example of medicalization. While earlier studies have pointed to the medicalization of women's bodies (Riessman, 1983; Martin, 1987; Riska, 2003), we now see aging men's bodies becoming medicalized as well.

This chapter examines three cases of the medicalization of masculinity: an as-yet lesser-known change, andropause; a commonly known bodily change, baldness; and erectile dysfunction. These cases raise interesting subtleties regarding the medicalization of masculinity. First, they point to a longstanding desire on the part of men, medical professionals, and entrepreneurs alike to achieve an old age that retains some of the essentially "masculine" and embodied qualities of youth and middle age—specifically, physical strength and energy, hirsutism, and sexual vitality. Thus, the medicalization of male aging, baldness, and sexual performance, while currently driven by the medical and pharmaceutical enterprises and accelerated by direct-to-consumer advertising, is also fueled by men's own concerns with their masculine identities, capacities, embodiments, and presentations. Second, the medicalization of these "conditions" occurred only partially by design; while the pharmaceutical industry was actively seeking treatments for these conditions, treatments emerged from research into other medical problems. Finally, two of these male "conditions" have been only partially medicalized. Although medical and pharmaceutical enterprises have offered treatments for andropause and baldness, there is no consensus about whether these constitute medical conditions, or—if they do—how their pathology is to be measured and assessed. Since the introduction of the drug Viagra (sildenafil citrate), erectile dysfunction has become increasingly medicalized. All three conditions exemplify the growing medicalization of men's bodies and masculinity.

GENDER AND MEDICALIZATION

Scholarly examinations of gender and medicalization, which have largely focused on the medicalization of women, have generally ignored the medicalization of men's lives. Some have argued that men are not as vulnerable to medicalization as are women (Riessman, 1983): the substantial literature on the medicalization of childbirth, premenstrual syndrome, menopause, and anorexia in women (Brumberg, 1988; Wertz and Wertz, 1989; Bell, 1990; Figert, 1995) clearly shows that more of women's life experiences are medicalized than men's. One of several reasons analysts typically give for women's vulnerability to medicalization is the traditional definition of a healthy body. On the one hand, Alan Petersen notes, "male bodies have been constructed through scientific and cultural practices as 'naturally' different from female bodies and the bodies of white, European, middle-class, heterosexual men have been constructed as the standard for measuring and evaluating other bodies" (1998: 41). On the other hand, Riessman (1983) suggests that women are more vulnerable to medicalization than are men because their physiological processes (menstruation, birth) are visible, their social roles expose them to medical scrutiny, and they are often in a subordinate position to men in the clinical domain. Riessman also argues that "routine experiences that are uniquely male remain largely unstudied by medical science and, consequently, are rarely treated by physicians as potentially pathological" (1983: 116).

However, while this may have been true when Riessman published her article in 1983, recent medical and scientific developments have contributed to the medicalization of aging male bodies. Although it is not my intent to refute the claims that Riessman and others have made about women and medicalization, I would like to make a case for the increasing medicalization of men and to broaden the understanding of medicalization as a truly gendered concept.[1] I first examine the scientific identification of the male hormone testosterone and the "discovery" of andropause, which is purportedly caused by an abnormal decrease of testosterone with age. Numerous medical testosterone-based treatments have been offered to alleviate this "disorder." Male hair loss, or baldness, is a common occurrence in aging men. Various elixirs and treatments have been introduced over the years, but in the past two decades new surgical and medical treatments have brought baldness further into the jurisdiction of medicine. Finally, the introduction of Viagra in 1998 led to an expansion and redefinition of male sexual performance and erectile dysfunction. Together these cases illustrate how medicine, expectations of masculinity, the physiology of aging, and the pharmaceutical industry contribute to the medicalization of male bodies.

AGING, MASCULINITY, AND THE BODY

Masculinity theorists, gender scholars, and anthropologists are concerned with the social processes and pressures that produce and constrain masculinity. The medicalization of men's aging bodies, through pressure to conform to certain standards of health, is one such source of constraint. A lack of discussion about the social factors that affect men's lives, including medical factors, contributes to an incomplete picture of contemporary masculinity.

In addition to masculinity, an analysis of medicalization that considers both age and the body as focal concerns can shed light on a number of intersecting sociological themes. First, through the lens of medicalization we can see a reflection of negative social beliefs about and fears of the aging process in men. We live in an ageist society in which the aging process is resisted and often feared. Instead of accepting the natural progression of the life course, we medicalize old age in an attempt to control it (Gullette, 1997; Marshall and Katz, 2002; Katz and Marshall, 2004). While researchers have paid attention to the aging process in women, particularly as it pertains to menopause (Friedan, 1993; Lock, 1993), aging men have been overlooked for several reasons. Thompson (1994) suggests that older men are invisible, in part because of the stigma that is placed on men as they disengage from traditional social roles and become more dependent. The longer life expectancy of women and reduced percentage of men in older cohorts may also play a role in this invisibility. In addition, feminist writers (e.g., Sontag, 1978) point to a double standard of aging, which suggests that men benefit from the aging process while women are stifled by it. As some have suggested, "Sociocultural constructions of femininity place considerable value on physical attractiveness and youth, and aging therefore moves women away from these cultural ideas" (Halliwell and Dittmar, 2003: 676). The growing market for testosterone, hair loss treatments, and Viagra-like drugs suggests that many men want to resist the aging process and may attempt to gain control of it by embracing its medicalization. Thus, as will become apparent later, men often collude in the medicalization of their capacities, characteristics, and functions.

Medicalization can provide insight into a burgeoning field: the sociocultural construction of the body (Turner, 1992; Gatens, 1996). A great deal of scholarship is dedicated to understanding the body as a social and cultural artifact (Scheper-Hughes and Lock, 1987; Sault, 1994). The body is the site where aging occurs, or, as Faircloth suggests, "the body visibly marks us as aging" (2003: 16). Understanding how medicine acts upon the aging body through definition, control, and surveillance helps create a fuller picture of the male experience of age. While aging can be understood on many levels, the body provides a salient frame of reference. Age is characterized by bodily change, and "the body [can] provide a key frame of reference for the male experience of health" (Watson, 2000: 87). By looking at "treatments" for the aging male body (testosterone, Propecia/Rogaine/hair transplants, and Viagra), we can understand how it becomes socioculturally constructed. As Mamo and Fishman suggest, "within the biomedicalization framework, medical technologies are part of programs and strategies of inscription that indicate the exercise of a rationalized, disciplining and regulating of bodies" (2001: 14). The infiltration of biomedicine into everyday life through commonly used medical treatments redefines "healthy" and "normal" in regard to bodily function. Men experience and understand their bodies differently if the aging process is constructed as pathological.

ANDROPAUSE: RUNNING ON EMPTY

Testosterone is the most intriguing of the male hormones. Physiologically, it is claimed, testosterone increases sex drive, musculature, aggressive behavior, hair growth, and other traits traditionally considered masculine (see Hoberman, 2005: 55–148). Healthy men maintain a relatively high (normal) level of testosterone throughout early and middle age, but bodily production of testosterone may naturally decline with advancing age. For the last century some physicians and other advocates have claimed that the age-related decline in testosterone levels results in a pathological condition, known as "andropause," that requires testosterone supplementation.

Currently, older men are being prescribed testosterone replacement therapy for a set of vague symptoms, often referred to as andropause, male menopause, the male climacteric, or androgen deficiency in aging men (ADAM). A recent Institute of Medicine report estimates that "more than 1.75 million prescriptions [for testosterone] were written in 2002, up from 648,000 in 1999" (Kolata, 2003). Despite the widespread use of testosterone replacement therapy, there is a dearth of information and clinical studies about its risks and benefits. Among many in the scientific community, including the National Institute on Aging and the National Cancer Institute of the National Institutes of Health, there is "growing concern about an increase in the use of testosterone by middle-aged and older men who have borderline testosterone levels—or even normal testosterone levels—in the absence of adequate scientific information" (Institute of Medicine, 2004: 1).

Uncertainty characterizes current medical knowledge both of the safety and efficacy of testosterone therapy and of the existence of a male menopause. This uncertainty is not new, as scientists and physicians have debated the existence of andropause for over a century. A brief exploration of the history of testosterone therapy and andropause reveals that the pharmaceutical industry, endocrinologists, the media, and men in general have promoted a medicopathological definition of aging. With its perceived potential to return the aging male body to a state of socially valued youthful vigor, testosterone has an almost magical attraction. Current media attention, the development of new pharmaceuticals, and the push to cast male aging and testosterone in medical terms are contributing to the further medicalization of the aging male body.

Historical Context for the Emergence of Testosterone Therapy

The discovery and isolation of testosterone undoubtedly contributed to the movement of male aging into the medical gaze. Although most of the scientific progress surrounding testosterone occurred during and after the nineteenth century, even before then "both folklore and medicine had explored the sources of maleness, seeking ways to promote strength, vitality, and potency" (Rothman and Rothman, 2003: 132). The medical definition of male aging had its origin in the work of scientists who pioneered the field of endocrinology. One of the most important ways that scientists made connections between testosterone and masculinity was through observations of castrated men. Because men without functioning testicles do not exhibit typical "male" attributes, the recognition that the testicles had some powerful effect on the male body predated the discovery of testosterone. Rothman and Rothman describe nineteenth-century common knowledge relating to the testicles and masculinity: "After all, as every farmer knew, the testes affected energy and muscularity; to castrate a rooster produced a capon—fatter, softer, and less active. To castrate an aggressive farm animal (a horse, dog, or bull) rendered him more docile and manageable. Indeed, popular lore recognized that men castrated whether by accident or on purpose . . . lost their manly characteristics" (2003: 132). Thus, according to this logic, an increase in the function of the testicles would amplify, enhance, or restore male traits from an undesirable level to a satisfactory one. Although they did not yet know that testosterone was produced in the testicles, many scientists, all of them male, applied this logic in exploring the testicles of a variety of animals.

It was not until 1889 that the endocrinologist Charles Edouard Brown Séquard made the connection between testosterone and aging. Brown Séquard completed a series of controversial experiments on himself. Motivated by a general feeling of malaise, weakness, and fatigue that had persisted for a few years, he injected himself ten times with "a solution composed of testicular blood, testicular extracts, and seminal fluids from dogs and guinea pigs" (Rothman and Rothman, 2003: 134). The results were spectacular and dramatic: Brown Séquard reported that he was now able to work long hours in the laboratory, "his muscle strength, as measured on a dynamometer, increased dramatically, his urinary jet stream was 25 percent longer, and his chronic constipation had disappeared" (Rothman and Rothman, 2003: 134). His findings sparked much interest in medical treatments for aging within both the scientific and lay communities. After a report of his presentation appeared in a French newspaper, "a geriatric horde descended on [his] laboratory at the Collège de France, demanding that he share his miracle potency restoring elixir with them" (Friedman, 2001: 251). Some physicians in France and the United States were quick to adopt Brown Séquard's formula in the hope of rejuvenating their aging male patients. Although Brown Séquard's results could never be reproduced and he was eventually denounced as a quack, he was the first person to connect male aging to a biological process and to suggest a medical remedy for it.

At the turn of the twentieth century, physiologists and early endocrinologists continued to be extremely interested in the science behind male physiology. Not surprisingly, researchers were more interested in masculinity than in fertility, as "they defined the male not so much by his ability to reproduce, but by his manliness" (Rothman and Rothman, 2003: 136). This concern with masculinity may have contributed to the medicalization of male aging and to the medicalized construction of andropause. In women, menopause is characterized by the cessation of fertility, a socially valued trait. This loss of fertility is considered the primary pathological event in the definition of menopause. Although men do not experience a decline in fertility when they age, they may notice a decrease in some of their allegedly masculine characteristics, such as libido, strength, and physical performance. Medicine, mirroring society, values these traits, and, as a result, provides a pathological explanation for their diminution or disappearance.

Endocrinologists prescribed a variety of testicular extracts to male patients; the scientific community then identified these extracts as useless when the male hormone was isolated in 1935. The accurate isolation of testosterone and the ability of pharmaceutical companies to synthesize it were accompanied by increased optimism within the medical scientific community. As Rothman and Rothman assert, "The newfound ability to produce the male hormone in the laboratory . . . sparked an even more zealous effort to establish its clinical uses" (2003: 151). Testosterone became a drug in search of a disease to treat. The excitement and increased optimism surrounding testosterone are particularly evident in medical journals following the 1935 discovery. Published articles illustrated the dramatic effects testosterone therapy could have on aging men. Many of these articles began by describing the patient before treatment as desperate. In an early issue of the *Journal of the American Medical Association (JAMA)*, for example, Dr. August Werner wrote, "In addition to markedly diminished sexual libido and inadequate penile erections, these patients, prior to treatment with testosterone propionate, were disturbed, anxious and broken in spirit" (1939: 1442). Patients who had not yet received testosterone therapy are described as pathetic, broken men, with little ability to function in a society that demanded so much of them (Kearns, 1939: 2257). By portraying the so-called male climacteric as a dire condition with potentially devastating consequences for male virility, physicians created a telling case for treatment. John Hoberman (2005: 115) suggests that the sexual conservatism of American physicians may have limited the clinical use of testosterone.

Early pharmaceutical companies had a great deal at stake with testosterone. The optimism and excitement that surrounded the isolation of testosterone were easily translated into marketing strategies that targeted physicians. Companies such as Schering, Oreton, and Ciba promoted the use of testosterone to the medical community in a variety of ways. In 1941 Schering produced a "clinical guide for physicians about male sex hormone therapy" (Rothman and Rothman, 2003: 157). Initially indicated for the treatment of sexual underdevelopment, hypogonadism, and testicular failure, Schering promoted testosterone therapy for the treatment of a broader scope of ailments, primarily the male climacteric. Such promotion of testosterone for male menopause was profit driven, as "sexual underdevelopment was too rare to constitute a substantial market" (Rothman and Rothman, 2003: 138). They thus worked to develop a wider market for testosterone, with advertisements (again targeted to physicians) portraying testosterone as a magic pill that could work wonders for middle-aged male patients. A 1924 advertisement from the *Endocrine Herald* promoted the use of Orchotine, a testicular extract. The advertisement proclaimed that Orchotine was "The Modern Treatment of Mental and Physical Sub Efficiency for Men." The text of the advertisement suggests to physicians that the use of this wonder drug will, beyond a doubt, correct the problems that afflict their aging male patients, such as fatigue and sexual apathy.

Andropause: Disease or Myth?

Andropause is not a clear-cut, easily identifiable, or definable condition. In a broad sense, andropause is defined as the age-related decline of testosterone levels in men that is accompanied by various symptoms, such as fatigue, lowered libido, and depression. The confusion surrounding the condition is "evident in the disputes over what to call it—andropause, veropause, male menopause, ADAM, and the male climacteric" (McKinlay and Gemmel, 2003). This conceptual confusion has existed for some time, as physicians and scientists have debated the use of each of these terms. A review of the current scientific literature reveals that it is misleading to describe the age-related decline of testosterone levels in men using terms like "andropause," "male menopause," or "the male climacteric" because, in Gooren's words, "terms like male menopause or andropause more or less suggest that, similarly to women, all men go through a profound decline of their androgen production from middle age on, but it should be stressed that the age-related decline of androgens in men follows a totally different pattern in comparison to the menopause" (2003: 350). In other words, "andropause" and "male menopause" are physiologically incorrect terms because, unlike women, men do not universally experience a cessation of gonadal function and reproductive capability (Hoberman, 2005: 141–43). In fact, "aging in healthy men is normally not accompanied by abrupt or drastic alterations of gonadal function, and androgen production as well as fertility can be largely preserved until very old age" (Nieschlag and Behre, 1998: 437–38).

Some in the medical community have suggested that the more accurate term "partial androgen deficiency in aging males" (PADAM) be used. This search for an accurate and scientific-sounding term is indicative of the process of medicalization, whereby a legitimate name for a condition promulgates its diagnosis.

While scientists agree that some men may experience a decrease in testosterone with age, the measure and meaning of testosterone levels remain contentious issues. Measuring testosterone levels is not straightforward: debates continue over whether the level of "free," bound, or total testosterone is the most significant measure (Stas et al., 2003). Concerns that testosterone levels can vary from hour to hour and that "periodic declines can occur in some otherwise normal men" (AACE, 2002: 442) fuel the debate as well. Thus, "there is currently no gold standard laboratory test" to determine testosterone levels (Tan and Culberson, 2003: 16), and no agreement as to what measurement to use to arrive at a diagnosis of andropause. The American Association of Clinical Endocrinologists (AACE) suggests, "An important research goal is to establish a consistent method for determining free testosterone levels and to verify the results so that these levels can be more widely used and trusted" (2002: 242). In short, standardizing ways to measure testosterone levels and creating agreement on what levels are considered abnormal will facilitate a diagnosis of andropause and contribute to increased rates of treatment—a crucial step in the medicalization of masculinity.

Moreover, while there is a basic understanding of testosterone decline and aging, scientists and clinicians know little about the mechanisms behind the decline and its connection to the physical manifestations of aging. It is clear that testosterone decreases with age, but whether this decline means that a man has a pathological condition such as andropause is not known. That professional societies such as the AACE are pushing for a resolution of diagnostic uncertainties, the acceptance of a standard laboratory analysis, and an accurate label to replace andropause is clear evidence that the medical and scientific communities are contributing to the medicalization of aging men's bodies. Indeed, despite the "humbling chasm of ignorance about testosterone therapy," as many as 1.5 million men are taking testosterone supplements (Vastag, 2003: 971). The availability of testosterone as a supplement in a convenient form will increase the chance that healthy men will use it to help them "treat" the symptoms of aging.[2]

Modern Pharmaceutical Companies and the Medicalization of Male Aging

Although testosterone therapy for the treatment of male menopause declined in popularity for most of the second half of the twentieth century, it never completely disappeared. Indeed, while the situation today is still somewhat ambiguous, the idea of a male menopause and the use of testosterone replacement therapy are reemerging, driven by technological advances made in the pharmaceutical realm and by the distribution of these drugs for an increasing range of male troubles. Both of these trends facilitate medicalization.

First, the mode of delivery for testosterone has evolved over the past few decades as pharmaceutical companies continue to search for treatments that are more convenient and attractive. With the availability of a highly effective and convenient form of the drug, more men are likely to participate in treatment. Oral preparations of testosterone, in the form of pills, are relatively easy to take. However, they are problematic because they do not maintain a constant level of the hormone in the body and may cause liver damage. Injections are uncomfortable for everyday use and "produce a sharp spike of the hormone, and then a fall, and these fluctuations are often accompanied by swings in mood, libido, and energy" (Groopman, 2002: 1). Patches, worn on the abdomen, back, thighs, or upper arm, maintain a steady level of the hormone but may be uncomfortable or fall off. The newest form of testosterone, a clear, odorless transdermal gel, can be rubbed into the shoulders once a day without any irritating effects. The main gel on the market today is AndroGel, a product of Unimed, an American division of the Belgian pharmaceutical company Solvay. The Food and Drug Administration (FDA) approved AndroGel in February 2000. Shortly after the FDA approval, Robert E. Dudley, president and CEO of Unimed, stated that "we believe that doctors and men who are waiting for a more convenient testosterone treatment will regard AndroGel as a very attractive alternative to existing testosterone replacement therapy" (*Doctor's Guide Global Edition*, 2000).

Second, while AndroGel is currently FDA approved only for well-defined conditions associated with hypogonadism, such as Klinefelter syndrome,[3] "pharmaceutical companies often obtain FDA approval of a new product for a niche population with a relatively rare disease, hoping to expand later to a larger and more profitable market" (Groopman, 2002: 3). Such "off-label" use of drugs is common medical practice and occurs when a physician prescribes a drug for conditions other than those for which the drug is approved. FDA regulations do not allow AndroGel to be advertised for any nonapproved uses, but pharmaceutical companies can use other avenues for promoting their product. For example, "they can run ads that 'raise awareness' of a condition without mentioning the proprietary therapy by name and they can align themselves with . . . well known physicians whose views are thought to have influence among their peers" (Groopman, 2002: 3). Unimed/Solvay has used both of these tactics to promote the use of AndroGel in aging men. Perhaps the most interesting technique is a menu option on AndroGel's website (www.andro gel.com) inviting the viewer to "Take the Low T Quiz." The questionnaire is derived from a 1997 "Androgen Deficiency in Aging Men Questionnaire"; the questions are vague and mirror many life changes that occur as men age. Questions such as "Have you noticed a recent deterioration in your ability to play sports?" or "Are you falling asleep after dinner?" hardly seem like clear medical symptoms, yet the implicit promotion of AndroGel turns these common life events into symptoms of a medical problem and suggests that a physician review the checklist.

The Allure of Testosterone

Although pharmaceutical companies promoting andropause have been prominent advocates for the medicalization of male aging, they are not alone. The promise of testosterone therapy has an almost magical allure for many people, including clinicians, their patients, and even the lay public. Testosterone is often portrayed as a miraculous substance, with amazing power to restore or enhance masculinity. The metaphors for testosterone in the public media illustrate the magical light in which the male hormone often is viewed. Men become complicit in their own medicalization with the promise that such treatments can produce astonishing results.

An advertisement for AndroGel from a recent issue of *Clinical Endocrinology* represents another way in which testosterone is framed to physicians and their male patients. The advertisement depicts a gas gauge with the arrow pointing to Empty. The text states, "Low sex drive? Fatigued? Depressed mood? These could be indicators that your testosterone is running on empty." Here, testosterone is depicted as fuel that can be used up; the male body does not naturally replace the material essential to sustaining its gender. Playing on the body-as-machine metaphor, with the brightly colored dial illustrating two poles, Empty and Full, the advertisement suggests that men can simply "fill up" with testosterone supplementation to regain sex drive, energy, and optimism—essentially masculine qualities. Testosterone supplementation is promoted as something that many men will need as part of the regular maintenance of their bodies. Instead of being depicted as a rare condition, andropause emerges as a mundane, typical, and predictable aspect of the daily life (and bodies) of men.

Testosterone therapy is also an attractive subject for the press. Different print sources have published stories with headlines like "Testosterone: Shot in the Arm for Aging Males" (*USA Today*, July 26, 2002) or "Are You Man Enough? Testosterone Can Make a Difference in Bed and at the Gym" (McLaughlin and Park, 2000). These pieces almost always begin with the personal story of a man who was tired at work, uninterested in sex with his wife, and failing on the football field/gym/squash court, whose life turned around after his physician prescribed testosterone. The article by McLaughlin and Park, published in *Time* magazine, is redolent with images of man as a sleek, powerful, and fast machine: "If you happen to be a man, the very idea is bound to appeal to your inner hood ornament, to that image of yourself as all wind-sheared edges and sunlit chrome" (2000: 58). This statement reflects a cultural preoccupation with reinvigorating the male body as a series of working parts that come together under the influence of "rocket fuel" (Friedman, 2001). Millions of aging male baby boomers compose an attractive market for both the media and pharmaceutical manufacturers (Friedan, 1993; Hepworth and Featherstone, 1998). The next decade will likely see testosterone replacement therapy become an important component of the medicalization of aging male bodies.

BALDNESS: PLUGS AND DRUGS

Losing one's hair or going bald is a common bodily occurrence that can cause anxiety among aging men. While remedies ranging from tonics and elixirs to bear grease have a long history, and medicine has long been concerned with hair loss, baldness has only recently begun to become medicalized. Although the medical profession is hesitant to call baldness a disease, the medicalization of baldness is gaining momentum in the light of new medical treatments for hair loss. Here too we see the invention and availability of medical therapies driving the process of medicalization.

A Brief Look at Historical Treatments for Baldness

Throughout history, men's concern with hair loss has given rise to an impressive range of remedies, potions, and concoctions to treat baldness. One of the first known written medical records, the Ebers Papyrus, dates back to 1500 B.C. and contains eleven recipes for the treatment of baldness. One recipe "advised the sufferer to apply a mixture of burned prickles of a hedgehog immersed in oil, fingernail scrapings, and a potpourri of honey, alabaster, and red ocher" (Segrave, 1996: 3). Baldness treatments were viewed in magical terms, and the treatment of baldness was left to alchemists who created concoctions that were shrouded in mystery. For example, in the sixteenth century A.D. the alchemist Paracelsus prescribed an elixir that purportedly contained "blood from women in childbirth, the blood of a murdered new born baby, and 'vipers' wine'" (W. Cooper, 1971: 153).

Until the late nineteenth century there was little medical interest in the cause of baldness or potential treatments for it: traditionally "the care of hair was left in the hands of charlatans, and treatments involved a mumbo jumbo of alchemy, magic, and superstition" (W. Cooper, 1971: 157). Also, because most remedies for baldness were ineffective, medicine had little to offer for the treatment of hair loss. However, the late nineteenth century saw the emergence of several medical theories about baldness. Physicians and scientists conceived a multitude of different causes of baldness, ranging from the logical to the bizarre—and, interestingly, none of them specifically gendered. One of the most popular theories was that hats caused baldness because "they compressed the circulation system, thus reducing nourishment to the hair" (Segrave, 1996: 14). Many physicians speculated on the hat theory, suggesting that the shape of the skull or the style of the hat were to blame. Accessing the new germ theory to present a pathological view of baldness, M. Sebouraud, a

French physiologist, announced at the 1897 meeting of the Dermatological Society of Paris that a microbe caused baldness. Medical journals warned that "combs should be boiled regularly and frequently, and under no circumstances should members of precociously bald families use other combs or brushes than their own, or allow them to be used on them, in barber shops, unless they are assured of their sterilization beforehand" (*JAMA* editorial, 1903: 249). Late-nineteenth-century dermatologists believed that irritating the scalp through blistering would cause hair regrowth. The procedure, known as vesication, "was believed to produce pooling of blood in the scalp, which provided more nourishment for the follicles there, causing hair regrowth" (Segrave, 1996: 52). Other treatments, no doubt equally painful, included vacuum caps and electric shock treatment.

Current Medical Understanding of Baldness

Despite or perhaps because of the quackery of the past, modern medicine has shown a keen interest in researching the causes of male-pattern baldness (referred to in the scientific literature as "androgenetic alopecia"). Although a Medline search we conducted for articles from 1985 to 2003 on androgenetic alopecia produced 356 citations, and although the term "androgenetic alopecia" evolved from the understanding that male baldness (alopecia) is dependent on male hormones (androgens) and genetics, there is disagreement over whether androgenetic alopecia is actually a disease. One textbook states, "The human species is not the only primate species in which baldness is a natural phenomenon associated with sexual maturity" (Dawber and Van Neste, 1995: 96). Other medical agents believe that "androgenetic alopecia becomes a medical problem only when the hair loss is subjectively seen as excessive, premature, and distressing" (Sinclair, 1998: 865), with some distinguishing between androgenetic alopecia and hair changes that accompany "natural" aging, known as senescent baldness. The dermatologist David Whiting writes, "The clinical and histologic evidence for senescent alopecia is not clear cut and is still disputed" (1998: 564). However, the ambivalence scientific writings express over the identity (or lack thereof) of male baldness as a distinct pathology coexists with the medicalization of male-pattern baldness as seen in the definition of androgenetic alopecia as an entity distinct from hair loss associated with "normal" aging.

Indeed, a science of hair loss has recently developed within this partially medicalized context: researchers have found that the male hormone dihydrotestosterone causes the hair follicle to produce the fine, unpigmented hair common in baldness. Growing evidence shows that male-pattern baldness runs in families and has a genetic basis: a gene called "sonic hedgehog" has been implicated in baldness. A *Sci-*

ence News article declares enthusiastically that "scientists suggest that a gene named after the combative [video game] character could prove a potent weapon in the battle against a fearsome foe: baldness" (1999: 283). A recent study published in *Nature Biotechnology* (Morris et al., 2004) suggests that stem cells may be helpful in curing baldness. Such findings have been significant in providing a medical basis for baldness and its treatment.

According to a definition mentioned earlier (Sinclair, 1998), androgenetic alopecia becomes a medical condition when hair loss is excessive. Determination of what constitutes excessive hair loss is subjective, yet medicine has created standards of hair loss through visual representations and quantitative means. Medical textbooks and journal articles contain diagrams that visually depict the progression of baldness. These diagrams, which are known as categorical classification systems, represent categories of increasing severity from mild to severe hair loss. Surgeons and dermatologists commonly use them, and this system "has become the standard of classification for hair restoration physicians" (Stough and Haber, 1996: 15).

Descriptions of baldness abound in medical terminology. Consider the following description, which corresponds to a Norwood level V classification: "*Type V.* The vertex region of alopecia remains separated from the frontotemporal region of alopecia. The separation is not as distinct as that in type IV because the band of hair across the crown is narrower and sparser. Both the vertex and frontotemporal areas of alopecia are larger than those in type IV" (Stough and Haber, 1996: 16). The language of this description is medically precise and does not assign subjective value to the phenomenon. Other diagnostic criteria exist, including measurements such as hair density, hair length, hair diameter, and cosmetically significant hair, defined as "a hair with a defined thickness and length, usually > 40mm and at least 3cm long" (Van Neste, 2002: 364). Medicine has attempted to quantify the exact length and diameter of a hair that would be considered attractive. Although the use of medical terms and measurements seems to remove any value judgments from the description of baldness, the standards are still subjective and influenced by sociocultural expectations. Even Van Neste, a clinical dermatologist, admits to the capriciousness of this measurement: "Fashion may . . . limit the application of the method depending on what hair style is desirable for the patient (e.g., a close hair cut is the currently popular style compared with longer hair in 1970)" (2002: 364).

Current Treatments for Baldness

Modern medical, surgical, and pharmaceutical technology has yielded treatments for baldness that differ from the snake oils of the past in their efficacy. They are currently the driving force in the medicalization of baldness. However, while effective, the drugs Rogaine and Propecia and hair transplant surgery are not miracle cures for baldness; they may be costly, painful, and for some men not useful. Despite such limitations, these treatments have been verified by the medical community, including the Food and Drug Administration, and are thus considered legitimate medical treatments. The cost of these treatments is significant, particularly for Rogaine and Propecia. Estimates from 1999 indicate that men spent $900 million on medical treatments (Rogaine, Propecia, and hair transplant surgery) for baldness; brand-name Rogaine costs $300 for a year's supply, and Propecia costs $600 (Scow, Nolte, and Shaughnessy, 1999). These expensive drugs are especially lucrative for pharmaceutical companies because the treatments must be continued indefinitely, or else the hair loss will resume. Meanwhile, hair transplants can cost anywhere from $2,000 to more than $10,000, depending on how many hairs are transplanted (Fischer, 1997). Here too the number of patients who will require repeat surgeries to maintain the transplant creates a lucrative market for hair restoration surgery.

Rogaine

The pharmaceutical company Upjohn was not seeking a baldness cure when it happened upon minoxidil, the active chemical in the drug Rogaine. In the mid-1960s, researchers found that minoxidil lowered heart rate. In 1979 the FDA approved the drug, known as Loniten, for the treatment of severe high blood pressure. Loniten was not expected to be a high profit drug, because it had a relatively specific target group. However, during clinical trials for hypertension, researchers noticed that one patient grew new hair on the top of his head. The growth was significant because it was dark, thick, terminal hair—the kind that is lost in baldness. When the media picked up research reports about this side effect of minoxidil, interested volunteers descended upon dermatologists and physicians in droves. An associate of Dr. Howard Baden, a Harvard researcher involved with early trials of minoxidil, says, "It wasn't even necessary to advertise for volunteers. All you have to do is whisper in the corridors that you're doing a study of male baldness and you get all the volunteers you want" (Segrave, 1996: 148). Clearly, the demand for an effective medical drug for male baldness was tremendous.

In the mid-1980s, even though the FDA had not approved the drug for treatment of baldness, many physicians were prescribing Loniten for their balding patients. This off-label use was so widespread that a 1986 survey estimated that "American dermatologists were prescribing topical minoxidil to over 100,000 patients per year" (Segrave, 1996: 153). It was clear that this growth was not due to an expanding hypertension market. In December 1985, Upjohn presented its newly researched baldness treatment to the FDA for approval. Approval was granted on August 18, 1988, once the company had modified its product information and changed the name of the drug to Rogaine (which the FDA felt was less misleading than the name originally proposed, Regain).[4]

The availability of Rogaine changed dramatically on February 12, 1996, when the FDA approved both the over-the-counter sale of the drug and the production of generic formulations of minoxidil. Determined to remain a leader in the hair growth market, Upjohn released a 5 percent stronger formula of Rogaine in 1997 and launched an advertising campaign emphasizing the strength of the new formula and of the men who use it. A 1999 advertisement features the tennis player John McEnroe promoting the "return" of Rogaine. The advertisement tells consumers that McEnroe "attacked" his bald spot and "beat" it. It also poses the question, "Is John the first man to snatch victory from the follicles of defeat? Far from it." Other Rogaine promotional materials use the slogan "stronger than heredity" and depict a bald father sitting next to his son with captions like "I love Dad. I'm just not in a rush to look like him." Rogaine is depicted as a drug that can give men power and control over a bodily change that was once perceived as inevitable. This is a seductive message, and one that reconfigures male aging as a vulnerable, though tenacious, foe.

Propecia

Rogaine's potential for profit was diminished when, on December 22, 1997, the FDA approved Merck's hair loss pill Propecia. Researchers stumbled upon the hair growth properties of the drug finasteride while it was being tested for use in men with enlarged prostates. The effectiveness of finasteride for preventing hair loss has been evaluated in three studies comprising a total of 1,879 men (Scow, Nolte, and Shaughnessy, 1999). Results are promising: the drug is effective in preventing baldness in the early stages of androgenetic alopecia. Current scientific understanding supports the early use of Propecia because in most cases of androgenetic alopecia, "prevention and maintenance are the most realistic therapeutic options" (Ramos e Silva, 2000: 729). Propecia works well for men who have just begun to notice signs of baldness, but it will not regrow hair. Because it cannot reverse significant hair loss, Propecia is not even technically a cure for baldness. To maintain the benefits of Propecia, men must take the medication for the rest of their lives, or they will revert back to the normal progression of balding.

Propecia targets self-conscious men who are troubled by their hair loss. Advertisements for the drug tell them that their impending baldness is preventable. Early Propecia advertisements depicted a man with a slight bald spot and a troubled, hopeless look on his face gazing into a bathroom mirror, seeing a reflection of himself as totally bald. The text of the advertisement reads, "If you think losing more hair is inevitable, think again." Another Propecia advertisement depicts a man with a bald spot staring at a dome. The text reads, "You don't need reminders about your hair loss. You need something to deal with it." Empowerment to attack hair loss and regain control is a central theme in both Rogaine and Propecia advertisements: even if a medical solution is not fully effective, the fact that one exists is enough to make men potentially empowered to do something about baldness. This is the attraction of drugs like Rogaine and Propecia, which contribute to medicalizing hair loss by providing men with medical treatments to conquer a troubling "disorder."

Surgical Treatments

The three surgical treatments for male-pattern baldness are transplants using a plug or graft technique, scalp reduction, and scalp flaps. I focus on only the first of these. As Bouhanna and Dardour assert, "The basic principle of the surgery of baldness consists in distributing the paucity of material as uniformly as possible" (2000: 29). Hair restoration techniques have limited effectiveness because baldness is a progressive condition: a transplant on a man in his thirties may look good at the time, but twenty years later his hair pattern may have changed significantly, rendering the cosmetic benefits of the transplant obsolete. Thus, although conceived of as a medical treatment for baldness, surgical procedures do not "cure" baldness but simply mask it. Textbooks and surgical atlases recognize this limitation. Marritt and Dzubow contend that "hair restoration" is a misnomer. "Sadly, hair restoration has nothing at all to do with the restorative process. Hair cannot be restored or resuscitated, only rearranged" (1996: 30).

Hair transplantation using plugs or grafts involves removing a section of the scalp from a part of the head that still has hair and sectioning this piece into "plugs" or "grafts" with a few follicles each. The plugs are then transplanted to the front of the scalp in an attempt to create a "natural" hairline. According to the surgical hair restoration literature, the creation of an "aesthetically pleasing" hairline is of utmost importance (Khan and Stough, 1996), as is "naturalness." A goal of this surgery is to make it appear as if it had never been done; one article even warns against "lowering the hairline to a position of youth . . . if the hairline is restored in a middle-aged person to the level of hair when they were 18 or so, it looks very unnatural" (Muiderman, 2001: 142). This paradox characterizes the entire field of hair transplant surgery. Overall, the procedures available today are only moderately effective, with side effects that include scarring, infection, and rejection of donor grafts. As a result, hair restoration surgery has had limited appeal as a medical treatment for baldness. The cutting edge of medical interventions for hair loss resides in pharmaceutical treatments.

Psychosocial Construction of Baldness

The psychological effects of baldness are one of the main justifications for treating hair loss as a disease. Medical textbooks and journal articles on the subject often devote a separate section to psychosocial concerns or the effect of hair loss on quality of life. As Valerie Randall asserts early on in her chapter on androgenetic alopecia, "In our youth-oriented culture, the association of hair loss with increasing age has negative connotations and, since hair plays such an important role in human social and sexual communication, male pattern baldness often causes marked psychological distress and reduction in the quality of life, despite not being life threatening or physically painful" (2000: 125). Indeed, some physicians cite the negative psychological correlates of baldness as the justification for medical treatment of hair loss. Emanuel Marritt, a hair restoration surgeon, sees this as his medical responsibility: "That 'simple office procedure' has, in reality, just handed me a life sentence of follicular responsibility. The weight of this awareness is not only humbling, it can be at times, simply overwhelming" (1996: 299). The exaggerated significance Marritt attaches to hair loss treatment reflects his awareness that as a surgeon he performs procedures more risky and invasive than what a dermatologist does when prescribing Propecia, but the viewpoint he expresses is an increasingly common one: hair loss is a serious problem worthy of medical intervention.

Given the Western cultural view of hair loss, it is not surprising that men may have negative views of baldness. A recent advertisement for Hershey's chocolate depicts the progression of baldness in a man accompanied by the slogan, "Change is bad." Although it has nothing to do with baldness therapy, the advertisement reinforces the view that bodily change due to age is an unwelcome stigma. Baldness, which often represents a loss of masculine traits, can affect male self-esteem. Psychological studies document the negative impact baldness can have on male mental health. Wells, Willmouth, and Russell (1995) found that hair loss in men is associated with depression, low self-esteem, neuroticism, introversion, and feelings of unattractiveness. There are, of course, cultural counterexamples of bald men. Actors like Yul Brenner and sports stars like Andre Agassi or Michael Jordan are not considered unattractive because they are bald. These men have embraced baldness and shaved their remaining hair. They have, in a sense, taken control of their hair loss. But these counterexamples stand in contrast to the general view of baldness as an undesirable condition, and one increasingly deemed appropriate for medical treatment.

ERECTILE DYSFUNCTION: THE ADVENT OF VIAGRA

The case of Viagra and the medicalization of erectile dysfunction has already been well documented (Carpiano, 2001; Mamo and Fishman, 2001; Loe, 2004), so I present here only the most important aspects of the medicalization of erectile dysfunction.

Male impotence has been recognized as a medical problem for many years. There is some evidence of medicalization in the Victorian era (Mumford, 1992), although its dominant framing throughout much of the twentieth century appears to have been as a psychogenic problem. In the 1990s the problem became redefined as "sexual dysfunction," and its treatment was promoted by urologists, the medical technology industry, mass media, and entrepreneurs (Tiefer, 1994). A consensus conference in 1992 officially renamed the problem "erectile dysfunction" (National Institutes on Health Consensus Development Panel on Impotence, 1993), highlighting its nature as a biogenic rather than psychogenic problem. Available medical treatments such as penile surgery, implants, and injections had mixed results (Tiefer, 1994).

In March 1998 the FDA approved Viagra (sildenafil citrate) as a treatment for erectile dysfunction. This drug was intended primarily for older men with erectile problems and for erectile dysfunction associated with prostate cancer, diabetes, or other medical problems (Loe, 2001). Although Viagra, like the pharmaceutical treatments for baldness, was a serendipitous discovery, it soon became the first noninvasive medical treatment for male sexual dysfunction (Loe, 2004). The medication operates by increasing the blood flow to the penis, allowing a man to achieve and sustain an erection when sexually aroused. Ingested orally, it takes effect in thirty to sixty minutes and can last from four to six hours.

A demand for a drug for erectile problems surely existed before Pfizer Pharmaceuticals, the manufacturer of Viagra, began advertising its new product. Estimates of the prevalence of erectile dysfunction range from 10–20 million men (Fabbri et al., 1997) to the suggestion that up to half of all American men are "sexually dysfunctional" (Laumann et al., 1999). Erectile difficulties affect not only men but their partners as well, and they are linked to powerful issues surrounding masculinity and sexual performance, making "erectile dysfunction central to masculine self esteem" (Tiefer, 1994: 370). Pfizer tapped into this vast potential market and shaped it by promoting sexual difficulties as a medical problem and Viagra as the solution.

With an aging population, a high prevalence of sexual dysfunction, and an even larger concern with insecurity about sexual performance, the potential American market was huge, with an even more extensive worldwide market. The initial advertising for Viagra was minimal (Carpiano, 2001), but Pfizer was soon marketing Viagra aggressively both to physicians and the general public. The direct-to-consumer ads included spokesmen as mainstream as former senator and presidential candidate Bob Dole, well-recognized athletes, and ordinary people, all testifying to the wonders of Viagra and how it had changed an important part of their lives. One typical ad featured baseball star Rafael Palmeiro with the words "I take batting practice"; it indicated both that vigorous athletes can take Viagra and that even stars might need some help in performance. Viagra became an official sponsor for Major League Baseball, for a car on the NASCAR circuit, and for Spanish-language soccer broadcasts. Thus, advertising expanded the market to include virtually any man who might consider himself as having some type of erectile or sexual problem.

Sales of Viagra were phenomenal. Physicians wrote 2.9 million prescriptions in the first three months of its availability; in the first year alone, more than 3 million men were treated with Viagra, translating into $1.5 billion in sales (Carpiano, 2001). Perhaps 200,000 prescriptions for Viagra are written weekly (Tuller, 2002), with untold more Viagra sold through the Internet and other outlets. In 2000, Viagra was ranked sixth in terms of both direct-to-consumer spending and sales, with a total of $89.5 million spent and $809 million in sales, and a 17 percent increase in use from 1999 to 2000 (NIHCM, 2001). By 2003, Viagra reached $1.7 billion in sales and was taken by 6 million men.

Viagra was a factor in the diagnostic expansion of sexual dysfunction and the increased medicalization of sexual performance (cf. chap. 3). Before Viagra, medical treatment was largely limited to major dysfunctions (e.g., as from prostate surgery). Now it included mild dysfunctions (e.g., occasional erectile problems) and could be used as an enhancement (Conrad and Potter, 2004), offering a "jump start" or extra strength for sexual encounters (Loe, 2001, 2004).

Viagra is not an inexpensive medication: it costs about $10 per pill. Within months of the FDA's approval of the drug, many large insurers (e.g., Kaiser Permanente and Aetna U.S. Healthcare) decided that they would not cover the drug, except at an extra cost to employers or individuals, while others (e.g., Blue Cross/Blue Shield plans in Indiana and California, Harvard Pilgrim Health Care, and the Defense Department's health plan) did cover the drug. However, many insurers who currently cover the drug limit the number of pills per month. For example, Tufts Health Plan (2002) covers four tablets every thirty days, and Blue Cross and Blue Shield of Texas (2003) covers eight tablets every thirty days. In Britain, however, the National Health Service covers Viagra only for sexual dysfunction related to conditions such as diabetes, prostate cancer, and renal failure (Michael Bury, University of London-Royal Holloway, personal communication).

The health insurance industry was involved in the debate over whether "sexual dysfunction" is a condition that requires medical intervention and whether Viagra should be covered by health insurance. The result of this debate was mixed insurance coverage for Viagra. In this case, the insurance industry attempted to counteract increased medicalization of male sexual dysfunction by restricting access to Viagra. However, individuals with a physician's prescription could of course purchase the drug on their own or through a range of Internet sites.

One important social benefit of the popularity and widespread use of Viagra is a reduction in the stigma of sexual dysfunction. Ads for Viagra in many mainstream locations and the mention of Viagra in everyday discussions have made sexual dysfunction and its treatment appear conventional and commonplace. This destigmatization has most likely increased the market for Viagra even further.

The success of Viagra and the subsequent extension of the concept of male sexual dysfunction has prompted other companies to enter and expand this market; these include pharmaceutical companies that are either developing new drugs like Levitra and Cialis to compete with Viagra (Conrad and Leiter, 2005) or seeking a "female Viagra" (Hartley, 2003; Moynihan, 2003). This trend (with men's maladies medicalized before women's problems) is the reverse of the usual order of gendered medicalization. Although the market for ED drugs shows some signs of plateauing (Berenson, 2005), given the aging of the baby boomers and the entrepreneurial pharmaceutical industry's increased promotion of "lifestyle" drugs marketed directly to consumers (Mamo and Fishman, 2001), the medicalization of sexual dysfunction will most likely continue to expand, at least for the foreseeable future.

MASCULINITY, MARKETS, AND MEDICALIZATION

Andropause and baldness represent aspects of aging male bodies that have become partially medicalized in recent years. In addition, the promotion of Viagra for erectile dysfunction has expanded from its initial focus on aging men to a much wider market with nearly all men as potential users. As new pharmaceuticals are developed and medical science comes to understand more about the physiological basis of aging, it is likely that medicalization will continue. Men and masculinity have often been omitted from analyses of medicalization, in part because of the belief that men are not as vulnerable to medical surveillance and control (e.g., monitoring and intervention for medical conditions) as women. But, as this chapter demonstrates, such a belief is no longer tenable.

Medicine has long been an avenue for women to resist the aging of their bodies and reclaim fading youthful features. Now this avenue is available and becoming increasingly appealing to men and a growing potential market. Youth and youthful manifestations of the body are paramount, as "contemporary expectations about health, fitness, and sexuality have pushed men to maintain youthful performance in all aspects of their lives" (Luciano, 2001: 204). Medical treatments can help men achieve this youthful appearance and performance.

While both andropause and baldness are medicalized aspects of aging male bodies, they have some contrasting features. Male testosterone levels decline as men age, but it is unclear what this means. Unlike menopause in women, andropause has no distinct markers or "symptoms." Although claims have been made regarding the benefits of testosterone replacement therapy, there is precious little evidence of any efficacy or improvement from such treatments. Baldness, on the other hand, is a distinct physiological condition, similar in some ways to a disease or disorder; it appears to have a genetic basis and creates what could be called a "bodily dysfunction." However, until recently it was not considered a medical disorder, nor were medical treatments available. With the advent of surgical and pharmaceutical treatments, though, hair loss has been increasingly medicalized; while not yet conceptualized as a disease, baldness is an actual bodily change that can be treated through medical interventions. In a sense, andropause has a medical name but unclear symptoms and no efficacious treatment. In contrast, baldness has clear symptoms and a range of medical treatments, some of which have achieved success.

The case of erectile dysfunction stands in contrast to andropause and baldness. While Viagra was first promoted for older men, Pfizer soon saw a much larger potential market. The pharmaceutical company extended its direct-to-consumer advertising to include virtually all men, and this expanded the definition of erectile dysfunction to include any erectile difficulties at any age. So the diagnosis "erectile dysfunction" expanded to occasional erectile problems or minimal problems with erection quality. "Ask your doctor if Viagra is right for you" became both a slogan and an invitation for all men to consider their erectile performance abilities. In a sense, Viagra became both a treatment for ED and a potential enhancement for sex (although pharmaceutical companies were initially reluctant to advertise the drug's benefits as such). With the introduction of Levitra and Cialis as competing products, advertisers specifically promoted these drugs to improve relationships and the quality of satisfaction (Conrad and Leiter, 2005). It should be noted, however, that along with medicalizing sexual performance, Viagra has also helped to destigmatize erectile dysfunction, making it a topic men and women could more freely discuss without embarrassment or shame.

In all cases, we see the infiltration of medicine into everyday life through labels or treatments that redefine "healthy" and "normal" male bodily function. Men experience and understand their bodies differently if the aging process is constructed in pathological terms. The maintenance of masculinity is often connected to the functioning of the male body. As body function declines, self-conceptions of masculinity may be imperiled. This may invite men to seek medical solutions to restore or retain the body's abilities, especially in Western culture wherein "all of us are encouraged to believe that our problem, aging, is natural, inevitable, awful, but controllable" (Gullette, 1997: 231).

This male anxiety about aging and masculinity, while not ubiquitous, is sufficiently common in American society to create a strong market for medical solutions. Given the growing number of aging baby boomers in our generally youth-oriented culture, it is not surprising that men are increasingly being seen as potential markets for medical solutions. The advent and promotion of products like AndroGel, Propecia/Rogaine, or Viagra/Levitra/Cialis may just be the beginning of a new medicalization of aging male bodies. The potential market expands when one considers that certain types of body maintenance and prevention must begin long before the onset of "old age" (Katz and Marshall, 2004). Pharmaceutical promotion of so-called lifestyle drugs, which "treat conditions understood not as life threatening, but rather as life limiting" (Mamo and Fishman, 2001: 16), is likely to be one of the greatest forces contributing to this form of medicalization. The combination of corporate promotion and consumer demand makes medical definitions and treatments of human conditions increasingly likely (Conrad and Leiter, 2004).

Concerns with aging and performance are propelling men to seek medical solutions for declining signs of masculinity. The perception of these physical changes as threats to traditional characteristics of manliness is not universal, but it seems to be increasing as pharmaceutical and medical entrepreneurs seek to establish markets, amplify male anxieties, and provide solutions to the problems of aging men. (See also Rosenfeld and Faircloth, 2006.) The medicalization of aging male bodies requires the joint action of men who seek solutions for a perceived decline in masculinity and the medical treatments that are offered to reinvigorate significant attributes of such masculinity. The partial medicalization of andropause and hair loss and the huge success of Viagra may be only the beginning. With baby boomers coming into their sixties, one may expect an expansion of medicalized categories and treatments for various ailments associated with aging men and masculinity.

CHAPTER THREE

Expansion

From Hyperactive Children to Adult ADHD

A wide range of new medical categories have emerged in the past four decades: attention-deficit/hyperactivity disorder, anorexia and eating disorders, chronic fatigue syndrome, repetitive strain injury, fibromyalgia, premenstrual syndrome, posttraumatic stress disorder, and multiple chemical sensitivity disorder. Many of these diagnoses have been promoted actively by individuals and their advocates, with some achieving substantial medical acceptance while others remain contested or controversial (M. Singer et al., 1984). By the close of the twentieth century, patients have become more engaged in their own treatment and more demanding in what they want from physicians (Guadagnoli and Ward, 1998), and less tolerant of mild symptoms and relatively benign problems (Barsky and Boros, 1995).

There are numerous reasons for seeking new medical diagnoses. Life's troubles are often confusing, distressing, debilitating, and difficult to understand. Michael Balint (1957) pointed out many years ago that a medical diagnosis transforms an "unorganized illness," an agglomeration of complaints and symptoms that may be unclear, unconnected, and mysterious, into an entity that is a more understandable "organized illness." As Broom and Woodward (1996) show with chronic fatigue syndrome, those with the disorder will often seek a diagnosis, which will both legitimate their troubles and provide them with an understanding of their problem. In some instances a diagnosis can be a kind of self-labeling that provides a new public identity as an individual having a particular illness or disorder. In other cases it may facilitate medical treatments that can have a substantial impact on individuals' lives. When these occur, it is hardly surprising to see individuals embracing medicalization.

The emergence of so many new medical categories raises the question of what happens with them over time. It is likely that some just become an established part of regular medical practice. Others may be challenged, disappear, or become vestigial from disuse, while others may expand in new ways. Medical diagnostic categories, perhaps especially psychiatric categories (Horwitz, 2002), are often fluid and subject to expansion or contraction. The expansion of established diagnoses is especially interesting, for it can occur almost unnoticed as a part of regular medical practice and at the same time expand the realm of medicalization in significant ways. To examine this phenomenon, we can find a similar process in the social constructionist frame for studying social problems.

"Domain expansion" describes a process by which definitions of social problems expand and become more inclusive (Best, 1990; Loseke, 1999). Domain expansion encompasses claims-making work that extends the definitional boundaries of an established social problem to include similar or related conditions. Joel Best (1990) examined the emerging definitions of child abuse and found that "by 1976, the issue encompassed a much broader array of conditions threatening children. The more general term 'child abuse' had replaced the earlier, narrower concept of 'battered child' and the even broader expression 'child abuse and neglect' had gained currency among professionals" (1990: 67). Valerie Jenness (1995) argued that activism by the gay and lesbian movement brought attention to the scope and consequences of anti-gay and lesbian violence. She suggests that domain expansion accompanied social movement growth and was key in reframing violence against gays and lesbians as a "hate crime" and as a specific public issue in the United States. While domain expansion need not always be linked to a social movement, the activities of champions and claims-makers are likely to be critical to the expansion of definitional boundaries.[1] Here I use the term "diagnostic expansion" in a similar fashion: how once a diagnosis is established, its definition, threshold, or boundaries can be expanded to include new or related problems or to incorporate additional populations beyond what were designated in the original diagnostic formulation.

This chapter focuses on the emergence of the diagnosis of attention-deficit/hyperactivity disorder (ADHD) in adults in the 1990s. How did hyperactivity, which was deemed largely a disorder of childhood, become adult ADHD? This research follows on my study of the medicalization of hyperactivity published in the 1970s (Conrad, 1975, 1976). Our interest here, however, is also to investigate this case as an example of how medicalized categories, once established, can expand to become broader and more inclusive. This category expansion is one means for increasing medicalization and provides us with an opportunity to explore how this aspect of medicalization operates. This chapter focuses on key claims and counterclaims made by mental health and medical professionals, as well as lay leaders, support groups, and conferences.[2] After reviewing the state of childhood hyperactivity as a medicalized diagnosis in the 1970s, I trace the emergence of "adult hyperactives" among those whose childhood symptoms persisted into adulthood, and then examine how this label was transformed into the category "ADHD adults." I show how lay, professional, and media claims helped establish the expanded diagnosis. I identify particular aspects of the social context that contributed to the rise of adult ADHD, and then outline some of the consequences of the medicalization of ADHD in adults and the social implications of expanding diagnostic categories.

THE DSM AS A CATEGORICAL TOUCHSTONE

Psychiatric diagnoses are historically and culturally situated. Certain diagnostic categories appear and disappear over time, reflecting and reinforcing particular ideologies within the "diagnostic project" (the professional legitimization of diagnoses) as well as within the larger social order (Cooksey and Brown, 1998: 550). As numerous researchers have noted, psychiatric diagnoses are not necessarily indicators of objective conditions but are a product of a negotiated interactive process influenced by sociopolitical factors (Kirk and Kutchins, 1992; Caplan, 1995; Kutchins and Kirk, 1997; Cooksey and Brown, 1998). Diagnoses related to behavior or involving cognitive symptoms are frequently contested or controversial, and thus diagnosis of "functional diseases" can "represent an implicitly negotiated solution to the problem of idiosyncratic suffering that is not explainable by specific pathology" (Aronowitz, 1998: 16).

Most psychiatric disorders gain legitimacy in the American Psychiatric Association's *Diagnostic and Statistical Manual of Mental Disorders* (DSM), the official guidebook for psychiatric diagnoses. Although the DSM does not contain all medical diagnoses, it can be seen as a repository of medicalized categories, especially those having to do with behavior. Despite its claims to psychiatric authority, it is not a scientific document but a "mix of social values, political compromise, scientific evidence and material for insurance forms" (Kutchins and Kirk, 1997: 11). As the authoritative voice of psychiatry, the DSM has been used as a mechanism to "secure psychiatric turf" (Kirk and Kutchins, 1992) and to sanction psychiatric categories.

The various revisions of the DSM have reflected distinct approaches taken by mental health professionals toward understanding human troubles as psychiatric conditions. In 1952 the original version of the DSM reflected the dominance of psychoanalytic thought and sought to "provide a broader set of labels, which would be inclusive of the whole society" (Cooksey and Brown, 1998: 530). A major shift in psychiatric thinking occurred with the publication of DSM-III in 1980, when the largely psychoanalytic orientation was abandoned and replaced with an avowedly biomedical and categorical approach to diagnosis. "The fundamental premise of

DSM-III was that different clusters of symptoms indicated distinct underlying diseases such as schizophrenia, depression, panic disorder and substance abuse" (Horwitz, 2002: 2). The "diagnostic project" was now heralded as a scientific endeavor, a claim that has increased with the publication of the DSM-IV (1994). This revision identifies nearly four hundred distinct medical diagnostic entities.

The DSM provides a useful touchstone for the sociological task of understanding how behaviors are defined medically, and especially for documenting how criteria for diagnosing a problem change over time and thorough various revised editions. In this way we can track some of the elasticity of a diagnosis such as ADHD.

HYPERACTIVITY IN THE 1970S

Although the roots of ADHD are often traced to early in the twentieth century (Goldman et al., 1998), it emerged as a diagnostic category only in the 1950s (see Conrad, 1975). Among several other diagnostic categories, it was termed at various times "minimal brain damage" or "minimal brain dysfunction" (MBD), "hyperactive syndrome," "hyperkinesis," and "hyperactive disorder of childhood." While there were slight differences among the categories, in practice they were interchangeable. The terms "hyperactivity" and "MBD" were most commonly used.

Beginning in 1968, the DSM-II identified "minimal brain damage" and other problems such as "hyperkinetic reaction" as a childhood disorder "characterized by overactivity, restlessness, distractibility, and short attention span, especially in young children; the behavior usually diminishes in adolescence" (APA, 1968: 50). The disorders were thus defined by both hyperactivity and inattention, two distinguishing features that would persist in various combinations throughout the next thirty years. (See also Stewart et al., 1966; Stewart, 1970; Wender, 1971.) Although this official classification clearly placed hyperactivity within the realm of childhood psychiatric illnesses, it also allowed for the possibility of its persistence into adolescence. For example, hyperactive behavior "usually" (but not always) "diminished" (though not necessarily disappeared) by the time the patient entered adolescence. Without solid evidence of biological causation, there nevertheless was an assumption of some type of organic pathology.

The most significant criterion for diagnosis was a child's behavior, especially at school. Hyperactive and disruptive behaviors were emphasized in identification (Conrad, 1976); thirty years later, behaviors are still the main criteria for identification (Conrad, 2006). The major treatments for hyperactivity were stimulant medications, especially Ritalin. During the 1960s the disorder became increasingly well known, in part as the result of publicity it received concerning controversies about drug treatment. By the mid-1970s it had become the most common childhood psychiatric problem (Gross and Wilson, 1974), and special clinics to identify and treat the disorder were established, although most children were diagnosed by their pediatrician or primary care physician.

While there were no methodologically sound epidemiological studies in the 1970s, it was widely estimated that 3–5 percent of elementary school students were hyperactive (occasionally estimates were as high as 10%); this is compared to the current Centers for Disease Control estimate of 7 percent of children aged 6–11 (CDC, 2002). Frequently mentioned estimates in the 1970s suggested that between 250,000 and 500,000 children were identified as hyperactive; current estimates are 4–8 million children in the United States (Conrad, 2006: xii). The disorder was believed to affect boys more often than girls, perhaps at a ratio of 9 to 1; this ratio has shifted to 3 to 1. Overall, hyperactivity was seen as fundamentally a disorder of childhood, typically identified in the early years of school, and most children were expected to "outgrow" it by adolescence (cf. Rafalovich, 2004).

THE EMERGENCE OF "ADULT HYPERACTIVES"

Beginning in the late 1970s, several cohort studies were published that followed children who had been originally diagnosed with hyperactivity a decade or more earlier and traced their development into adulthood. These studies established that the symptoms of some hyperactive children persisted into adolescence and even into adulthood. Thus emerged the notion of what we can call "adult hyperactives"—hyperactive children who did not "outgrow" their symptoms and still manifested some problems as adults.

Gabrielle Weiss and colleagues (1979) followed 75 hyperactive children and 45 matched controls for fifteen years. They found that clear symptoms persisted for many hyperactive children into adulthood; 66 percent had at least one symptom (G. Weiss and Hechtman, 1986). Most notable was the persistence of restlessness and poor concentration. Despite criticisms that only 60 percent of the children were followed into adulthood, the study remains widely cited (and mis-cited).[3] A second prospective study found that 31 percent were still diagnosable as hyperactive in late adolescence (Gittleman et al., 1985; see also Mannuzza et al., 1991, 1998). A follow-up at young adulthood, however, showed a significant decrease of symptoms, to about one-third the rate reported by Weiss. The media has tended to focus on the higher prevalence rates reported in the Weiss data.

Following the publication of these seminal studies, other researchers (e.g., Biederman et al., 1996) investigated the persistence of symptoms into adulthood to further identify what they believed to be confounding factors (such as comorbidity with other disorders). These studies reflect the dominant thinking of the late 1980s: any diagnosis of attention-deficit disorder (or ADD, as the disorder was renamed) was found only among adults whose disorder persisted from childhood and thus was *not* a disorder that was either "missed" during childhood or was of adult onset. All ADD adults were hyperactive children who had grown up.

The 1980 update, DSM-III, both reflected and facilitated an interest in hyperactivity beyond childhood.[4] First, in line with the general trend in DSM-III to define disorders by symptoms rather than etiology, the updated manual reclassified the disorder according to its primary symptoms: either hyperactivity *or* inattention. Thus the diagnosis focused on *attention* deficits with two major subtypes: attention-deficit disorder with hyperactivity and attention-deficit disorder without hyperactivity (deemed the less severe of the two categories). The symptoms were focused largely on children's activities (e.g., "runs about or climbs on things excessively," "frequently calls out in class," or "has difficulty concentrating on schoolwork or other tasks requiring sustained attention"). To be diagnosed, patients needed to exhibit symptoms before age 7.

Second, the range of behaviors included within the official diagnosis became more comprehensive. Some symptoms were related to school-based behavior such as "frequently calls out in class," whereas others were more interpersonal and ephemeral in nature (e.g., "often acts before thinking" or "is easily distracted"). These changes in the diagnostic category meant that individuals who may not have "qualified" for a diagnosis of hyperkinetic reaction or minimal brain damage under DSM-II could now be thought of as having ADD under DSM-III. Both subtypes of ADD permitted courses of the disorder in which "all symptoms persist into adolescence or adulthood" or in which "hyperactivity disappears but other signs persist into adolescence or adulthood" (APA, 1980: 42). Thus, the DSM-III definition expanded the diagnostic criteria in terms of necessary "symptoms" while allowing for the possibility for persistence into adulthood.

THE DEVELOPMENT OF "ADHD ADULTS"

In the 1987 revision, the DSM-III-R, ADD was renamed "attention-deficit/hyperactivity disorder" (ADHD) to reassert the condition of hyperactivity as one possible, but not mandated, symptom of the disorder. ADHD enabled children who were hyperactive and impulsive but less inattentive to meet the diagnostic criteria. More than 50 percent more children received the ADHD diagnosis under these criteria (Newcorn et al., 1989). The revised diagnostic criteria did not refer to the disorder in adulthood but opened the door slightly for an expanded definition beyond "adult hyperactives" to "ADHD adults" who had no childhood diagnosis. For example, the environment in which ADHD symptoms occurred had expanded to the workplace: "In the classroom or workplace, inattention or impulsiveness are evidenced" (APA, 1987: 50). There was less emphasis on school-aged behaviors: "frequently calls out in class" (DSM-III) became "often blurts out answers to questions before they have been completed." Nevertheless, the criterion of exhibiting symptoms before age 7 was retained, and although the revision obliquely acknowledged the possibility of postchildhood ADHD, adult ADHD was not highlighted in the manual.

Early Claims

In this same year that the DSM-III-R was published, two publications aimed at lay readers heralded a new category of "ADHD adults"—adults who had not been diagnosed as children but had had symptoms. Although later claims would be made by those who could not trace their symptoms to their youth, these early claims were made either by or for those who retrospectively could identify signs of ADHD in their childhood.

In 1987, Paul Wender, a longtime hyperactivity researcher, published a book that examined hyperactivity throughout the life span. Although the book was entitled *The Hyperactive Child, Adolescent, and Adult*, only one chapter described adults with ADHD symptoms. Nonetheless, the book targeted a lay audience and would be cited frequently in subsequent years.

The same year, Frank Wolkenberg (1987), a freelance photographer and picture editor, wrote a first-person account in the *New York Times Magazine* about his discovery that he had ADHD despite his apparently successful life. When he sought treatment for depression and suicidal ideation, he was diagnosed with ADHD by a psychologist whose specialty was learning disorders. Wolkenberg then began reinterpreting several clues early in his life (e.g., impulsivity, distractibility, disorganization, and emotional volatility) as signs of the disorder. This highly visible testimony of someone not previously diagnosed with ADHD as a child put the idea of "ADHD adults" into the public realm. No one had diagnosed him as hyperactive as a child, yet now he was attributing "seemingly inexplicable failures . . . all unnecessary and many inexcusable" (p. 62) to ADHD. He suggested that it was a neurobiological dysfunction "of genetic origin," thus attributing his life problems to a chemical imbalance.

As the notion of ADHD in adulthood was filtering into the public awareness, the psychiatric profession was also turning attention to this new problem. Clinics for adults with ADHD were established at Wayne State University in 1989 and two years later at the University of Massachusetts in Worcester (Jaffe, 1995).

In 1990, Dr. Alan Zametkin of the National Institute of Mental Health and several of his colleagues published an often-cited article in the *New England Journal of Medicine*. Using positron-emission tomography (PET) scanning to measure brain metabolism, Zametkin demonstrated different levels of brain activity in individuals with ADHD compared with those without the disorder; these findings provided new evidence for a biologic basis for ADHD. Because of the risks inherent in research involving radiologic images, the researchers used adult subjects who had childhood histories of hyperactivity and were biological parents of hyperactive children. Although this was not Zametkin's intention, his work became one of the key professional sources cited by others to demonstrate the presence of ADHD in adults (e.g., Bartlett, 1990; *Newsweek*, December 3, 1990), because it appeared to bolster claims that ADHD could persist into or develop during adulthood.[5] While the study made national headlines, additional follow-up studies that did not confirm the strength of the initial study's findings received no widespread publicity from the professional and lay press.[6]

Adult ADHD in the Public Sphere

Writing about ADHD as a disorder in adults has been increasing in the professional literature for years. As can be seen in table 3.1, by the mid-1980s there were more than forty articles in the medical literature and about a dozen in the psychological literature published per year (with some overlap). Many of these articles were minor, and nearly all dealt with the persistence of symptoms in hyperactive children as they reached adulthood. The issue of "ADHD adults" per se did not reach the popular media until the 1990s (see table 3.1). But the idea that adults could have ADHD did spread with the help of a moderate but growing number of articles in a variety of media.

In the early 1990s, several books written for a popular audience looking specifically at ADHD adults were published. Psychologist Lynn Weiss (1992) identified her adult subjects as those who were diagnosable with ADHD, not merely grown-up hyperactive children having remnants of the symptoms carried over from an earlier condition. Another popular book quickly followed with the provocative title of *"You Mean I'm Not Lazy, Stupid, or Crazy?!"* (Kelly and Ramundo, 1993). This book emphasized the shift in responsibility that a diagnosis of adult ADHD can bring. Thom Hartmann (1994), writing in a somewhat esoteric but essentially sociobiological frame, associated ADHD with an evolutionary adaptation to the social environment. He likened those with ADHD to hunters (who are nomadic, scanning the environment for sustenance, seeking of sensation, reacting quickly and decisively) adapting

TABLE 3.1

*Adult ADHD in the Professional and Lay Media: Mean Articles Per Year,
1975–1999, in Five-Year Intervals*

| Years | Professional Media | | Lay Media (Academic Universe) | | |
	Medline	PsycINFO	Wire Services	NE Regional	Magazines
1975–1979	34.4	3.4	0	0	0
1980–1984	41.6	7.6	0	0	0
1985–1989	43.6	11.4	0	0.2	0.4
1990–1994	50.0	13.8	5.8	6.0	0.4
1995–1999	95.6	42.6	25.2	28.6	32.2

Notes: For this table, I do not distinguish between articles on "adult hyperactives" and "ADHD adults."

Search criteria for professional media: adult and (ADHD or "attention deficit disorder" or "attention-deficit/hyperactivity disorder" or hyperkinesis).

Search criteria for lay media: in-text search for "attention deficit disorder or ADHD or hyperkinesis" and search in headline or lead paragraph for "adult."

Lay media sources include wire services (e.g., Associated Press, United Press International), New England regional newspapers (e.g., *Boston Globe, New York Times*), and popular magazines (e.g., *Ladies' Home Journal, Newsweek*).

to a more modern farming community (which requires greater stability and focus). This hypothesis, by its nature, supports the notion of ADHD in adults.

Further support came from the television news media reports on the spread of ADHD in adults. Major news shows put their own spin on the prevalence of the disorder. For example, on *20/20*, Catherine Crier attributed ADHD to a "biologic disorder of the brain" in adults (September 2, 1994). Dr. Timothy Johnson on *Good Morning America* (March 28, 1994) was quoted as saying that experts estimate as many as 10 million adult Americans may have ADHD (reported in Vatz and Weinberg, 1997: 77). The new face of the disorder was not limited to hyperactive children grown up but included a new group of "ADHD adults" who came to reinterpret their current and previous behavioral problems in light of an ADHD diagnosis.

The message was reiterated in popular magazines. A feature article in *Newsweek*, for example, described a 38-year-old security guard who had held more than 128 jobs since leaving college after having been enrolled in the academic institution for thirteen years (Cowley and Ramo, 1993). He finally "received a diagnosis that changed his life" at the adult ADHD clinic at the University of Massachusetts in Worcester. Similarly, an article in *Ladies' Home Journal* (Stich, 1993) described a husband who was fired from job after job, constantly interrupted his wife, and forgot details of conversations. Then, "two years ago, the Pearsons discovered there was a medical reason for Chuck's problems. After their son was diagnosed with attention deficit disorder (ADD) . . . they learned Chuck also had the condition" (p. 74). The article does not mention the fact that Chuck, who was diagnosed at age 54, also went on to found the Adult Attention Deficit Foundation, which acts as a clearinghouse for information about adult ADHD (Wallis, 1994: 47).

Adult ADHD was given a great boost in 1994 with the publication of the best-selling book *Driven to Distraction* by Edward Hallowell and John Ratey (1994), two psychiatrists with prestigious organizational affiliations. Hallowell offered his own experience as the springboard for the book: although successful as a medical student and later as a practicing psychiatrist, he came to believe that he had ADHD. Ratey also stated that he had ADHD. Their book has become a crucial touchstone among the lay public. Using their clinical experience as the basis for their book, Hallowell and Ratey argue that ADHD takes various forms. Based upon their clinical experience, they propose "suggested diagnostic criteria for attention deficit disorder in adults" (p. 76). These criteria recognize the disorder without hyperactivity. Hallowell and Ratey present thirteen subtypes of the disorder, a set of "suggested diagnostic criteria," and a one-hundred-question test (with elusive criteria)[7] to enable readers to assess whether they need to seek evaluation for ADHD. The authors urge readers not to self-diagnose but to seek professional assessment. Neither Hallowell nor Ratey is a hyperactivity researcher: Ratey published only one article in the topic in a professional journal (Ratey et al., 1992) and Hallowell none. Both remain active in promoting their work in public circles. Their affiliation with Harvard Medical School gave them some academic legitimacy, but they came to the area of ADHD adults more as professional advocates than as scientific researchers. In a sense, they are moral entrepreneurs for the adult diagnosis (Leffers, 1997).

The cover of July 18, 1994, *Time* magazine issued a clarion call for adults with ADHD: "Disorganized? Distracted? Discombobulated? Doctors Say you Might Have ATTENTION DEFICIT DISORDER. It's not just kids who have it." The nine-page article disseminated the criteria and possibilities of ADHD in adults to a wide audience, and it speculated that Ben Franklin, Winston Churchill, Albert Einstein, and Bill Clinton may have had the disorder (Wallis, 1994).

Over the years a number of organizational stakeholders emerged to focus on ADHD in children; these parent and advocacy groups included those involved in the learning disabilities movement (Erchak and Rosenfeld, 1989). The largest ADHD support group, Children and Adults with Attention-Deficit/Hyperactivity Disorder (CHADD), has grown significantly over the last decade and owes much of its growth to its adult membership, specifically those adult members with ADHD. In its activities as well as its framing of ADHD, the organization has helped expand the categorization to include adults. In 1990 the parent organization sponsored a national meeting that featured three adults with ADD and four professionals as speakers (Jaffe, 1995). In 1993 the organization added the "and adults" to its name to reflect its broadened focus. In May 1993 a CHADD-sponsored national conference entitled "The Changing World of Adults with ADD" attracted participants from thirty states and two Canadian provinces. The organization now sees education and support of adults with ADHD as part of its core mission. For example, on its web page the organization proclaims, "AD/HD is a lifespan disorder that affects individuals at all ages" (www .help4adhd.org/faqs.cfm#faq4). In addition to lobbying for educational services for children, CHADD advocates for legislation that provides workplace protection for adults with ADHD.[8] In all official publications and communications, CHADD has positioned ADHD as a medical condition, a "neurobiological disorder," rather than as a psychiatric or behavior disorder (Diller, 1997: 130; www.chadd.org), so it can be perceived as having a more legitimate stake in disability entitlements.

CHADD has played a significant role in bringing the lay and professional claims-makers together to promote better understanding, acceptance, and treatment of ADHD (Leffers, 1997). CHADD promotes the existence of adult ADHD to the public and legitimates the disorder for individuals almost as much as the actual diagnosis does. Like groups that represent individuals with other controversial illnesses (see, e.g., Kroll-Smith and Floyd, 1997), the organization is both a haven and an advocate for those who believe they have the disorder.

Another organizational stakeholder is the pharmaceutical firm Ciba-Geigy, which manufactures Ritalin (methylphenidate), the drug most widely prescribed for treating ADHD. Ciba-Geigy has long been involved in framing hyperactivity and now ADHD as a medical disorder (Conrad, 1975; Schrag and Divoky, 1976). As early as 1971, Ritalin provided as much as 15 percent of Ciba's gross profits (Conrad, 1976: 16). While the original patent on the drug has long since expired and methylphenidate is available in generic formulations, Ritalin is still the most commonly prescribed medication for ADHD (Arnst, 1999) and one of the three most commonly prescribed stimulants (S. Ballard et al., 1997). The amount of methylphenidate manufactured increased sharply in the 1990s. From 1990 through 1999, the production of methylphenidate in the United States grew by 700 percent (*New York Times*, January 18, 1999).[9] One national survey of physicians' diagnoses, based on 1993 data, found that of the 1.8 million persons receiving medications for ADHD, 1.3 million were taking methylphenidate (cited in Diller, 1996: 12). Other sources have variously estimated that 2.6 million children (Guistolise, 1998) and 729,000 adults received prescriptions for Ritalin (Breggin, 1998: 160). The potential market, with 3 million children and 4 million adults in the United States diagnosed with

ADHD (Arnst, 1999), has untapped pockets.[10] By redefining ADHD as a lifetime disorder, the potential exists for keeping children and adults on medication indefinitely. A 1999 review article noted, "The eightfold increase in the use of stimulants in the United States over the past decade stems from several factors, including the continuation of treatment from childhood into adolescence and the treatment of adults" (Zametkin and Ernst, 1999: 45). Prescriptions for ADHD medications for people aged 19 years or older "increased by 90 percent between March 2002 and June 2005," with adults accounting for approximately one-third of all prescriptions for these drugs (Okie, 2006: 2638). While it is difficult to assess accurately what proportion of this huge increase in stimulant medication use is for adults with ADHD, the proportion is likely to be substantial.

These organizational stakeholders—both advocacy groups and pharmaceutical companies—have worked both independently and in consort. Ciba-Geigy reportedly has provided significant financial assistance through a variety of support mechanisms that assist adults with ADHD, including the support group CHADD and a video produced for the Office of Special Education Programs (OSEP) (Diller, 1996). In 1995 the *Merrow Report*, a public radio talk show, reported that CHADD received significant financial contributions from Ciba-Geigy (PBS, 1995). The public outcry and media attention questioned the neutrality of this group. According to CHADD's 2004–5 Annual Report, the organization received 22 percent of its nearly $4.5 million revenue from pharmaceutical companies through unrestricted educational grants (www.chadd.org/AM/Template.cfm?Section=Reports1&Template=/CM/ContentDisplay.cfm&ContentID=1771).

Diagnostic Institutionalization

By 1994, the DSM-IV reflected the growing consensus that adults could be diagnosed with ADHD, provided they had exhibited symptoms as children before the age of 7. Two (out of the five) diagnostic criteria clearly were relevant to adults. First, the DSM-IV required that "some impairment must occur in at least 2 settings." While for children these settings usually mean school and home, the range of settings may be greater for adults and include home, school, work, and other vocational or recreational settings. Second, and related, "there must be clear evidence of interference with developmentally appropriate social, academic or occupational functioning." The inclusion of work environments in the criteria section of the manual reflected the central and relatively uncontroversial position the diagnosis of ADHD in adults now occupied.[11]

The new definition allowed for more variations of symptomatic behavior across and within settings. "It is very unusual for an individual to display the same level of dysfunction in all settings or within the same setting at all times" (APA, 1994: 79). Adults who might be quite successful at work but highly inattentive in particular interpersonal relationships and recreational activities could now be diagnosed with ADHD. As the more expansive criteria in the DSM-IV have gained acceptance among mental health professionals, some have advocated eliminating the requirement that adults be able to retrospectively reconstruct a history of ADHD (Barkley and Biederman, 1997). This would permit even greater expansion of the adult ADHD category.

Reports from the American Medical Association (AMA) and the National Institutes of Health (NIH) have supported an expanded ADHD diagnosis.

In 1997 the Council on Scientific Affairs of the AMA issued recommendations for treating ADHD. These recommendations were published in the *Journal of the American Medical Association* (April 8, 1998): "The criteria of what constitutes ADHD in children have broadened, and there is a growing appreciation of the persistence of ADHD into adolescence and adulthood. As a result, more children (especially girls), adolescents, and adults are being diagnosed and treated with stimulant medication, and children are being treated for longer periods of time" (Goldman et al., 1998: 1100). The report concluded that there was "little evidence of widespread overdiagnosis or misdiagnosis of ADHD or of widespread overprescription of methylphenidate by physicians" (p. 1100). In November 1998 the NIH convened a Consensus Conference on the Diagnosis and Treatment of Attention Deficit Hyperactivity. While little new emerged from the conference, two papers explicitly focused on adults with ADHD. Overall, the conference report affirmed the validity of ADHD, although it recognized scientific controversies, the need for more basic and longitudinal research, and a lack of consensus on optimal treatment (www.consensus.nih.gov/1998/1998AttentionDefi citHyperactivityDisorder110html.htm).

Further institutional support for the ADHD diagnosis in adults has come from prestigious professional publications. A lead editorial in the *American Journal of Psychiatry* (Shaffer, 1994) and major review articles in *New England Journal of Medicine* (Elia et al., 1999; Zametkin and Ernst, 1999), all of which included discussions of ADHD in adults, signaled the acceptance of the diagnostic category in medical circles.

By 1994 the clinical diagnosis of ADHD, which had expanded to include adolescence and adulthood, had become institutionalized in psychiatry and medicine. One longtime researcher called it "the most common chronic undiagnosed psychiatric disorder in adults" (Wender, 1998: 761).

Self-Diagnosis

One of the starkest contrasts to the earlier history of ADHD with children is the vast amount of self-diagnosis of ADHD among adults. Virtually all children are referred to physician by parents or schools (Conrad, 1976; Rafalovich, 2004). In contrast, among adults, self-referrals are the norm, and many patients come to physicians apparently seeking an ADHD diagnosis. Frequently, adults who encounter a description of the disorder sense that "this is me" and go on to seek professional confirmation of their new identity. Another common path to self-diagnosis occurs when parents bring a child to a physician for treatment and remark, "I was the same when I was a kid," and thus they begin to see themselves and their own difficulties through the lens of ADHD. While this trend appears to have been precipitated by some of the popular press (e.g., Hallowell and Ratey, 1994), it continues with legitimization provided by support groups designed for adults with ADHD such as CHADD.

Anecdotes in the popular literature suggest that adults who self-diagnose may recognize their condition in a popular media article or book. Hallowell and Ratey describe one woman who noted, "My husband showed me this article in the paper" (1994: 26). Comments on Internet sites state that one of the books on adult ADHD led individuals to physicians for a diagnosis. Diller (1997) relates that one of his patients came to self-diagnosis after reading *Driven to Distraction*. Diller points out that while the physician who is presented with such a self-diagnosed patient may have difficulty establishing the existence of symptoms in the person's childhood (as opposed to a checklist of symptoms absorbed through reading), the self-diagnosis itself becomes an element that the professional diagnosis must take into account. One psychiatrist wrote to a colleague, "Adult ADHD has now become the foremost *self-diagnosed* condition in my practice. I fear that the condition allows a patient to find a biological cause, that is not always reasonable, for job failure, divorce, poor motivation, lack of success, and chronic depression" (Shaffer, 1994: 638).

Diagnosis-seeking behavior is an integral feature of the emergence of adult ADHD. This kind of self-labeling, information exchange, and pursuit of diagnosis fuels the social engine medicalizing certain adult troubles. Without it, the spread of adult ADHD would be seriously limited.

Critics, Skeptics, and Counterclaims

Even with well-established diagnoses such as ADHD in children, there may be skeptics and critics who dismiss the validity of the diagnoses, criticize overdiagnosis, or enumerate the dangers of pharmacological treatment. Although such attempts to reign in medicalization have had little impact on adult ADHD, they remain a reservoir of counterclaims that could affect diagnostic expansion.

Some therapists who treat those with ADHD believe that the diagnosis is becoming too prevalent: "Certainly, some people diagnosed with ADHD are neurologically impaired and need medication. But the disorder is also being named as the culprit for all sorts of abuses, hypocrisies, neglects and other societal ills that have nothing to do with ADHD" (Bromfield, 1996: 32). Alan Zametkin, a leading researcher on ADHD, has become quite critical of what he has called "a cottage industry of adult ADD" (Kolata, 1996).

In the late 1980s the Church of Scientology launched a major media campaign against the use of Ritalin with children. Although the controversial church remained an outsider in the debate, for several years its members voiced public criticism about ADHD (Leffers, 1997). Furthermore, a number of popular books critical of the "epidemic" of ADHD and Ritalin use have been published: *Running on Ritalin* (Diller, 1997), *Ritalin Nation* (DeGrandpre, 1999), and *Talking Back to Ritalin* (Breggin, 1998). While most of these books focused their criticism on the diagnosis and pharmacological treatment of children, they expressed some skepticism about the disorder in general.

The popular media, which had been actively involved in publicizing the prevalence of the disorder among adults in 1993 and 1994, became more critical in subsequent years. Leading the challenge was a cover story in *Time* magazine (Wallis, 1994); the synopsis banner read, "Doctors Say Huge Numbers of Kids and Adults Have Attention Deficit Disorder. Is It for Real?" The television program *60 Minutes* (December 10, 1995) produced segments that highlighted the absence of a definitive test for ADHD. Other major news shows focused on controversies about the subjectivity of ADHD diagnoses and the overprescription of Ritalin (e.g., the *Today* show on October 24, 1995; CNN on November 2, 1995; 20/20 on December 20, 1995; and *ABC Evening News* on March 28, 1996—reported in Vatz and Weinberg, 1997). Recently, concern has been voiced about an increased cardiovascular risk from taking ADHD drugs (Nissen, 2006).

Most of the criticism has been about the overdiagnosis and treatment of children. Even in this context, a steady number of articles have supported treatment of the disorder (e.g., Gladwell, 1999). Only a small amount of the criticism has been directed against notions of adult ADHD. Ironically, though, controversy about ADHD raises public awareness and increases the diffusion of information about the disorder, which can indirectly contribute to diagnostic expansion.

THE SOCIAL CONTEXT FOR THE RISE OF ADULT ADHD

The expansion of the hyperactivity diagnosis to adults is not primarily the result of new scientific discoveries about the biomedical nature of the disorder. While many studies have indicated that symptoms in children diagnosed with ADHD could persist beyond childhood, the studies have also showed that this occurred in perhaps a third of the cases (G. Weiss et al., 1979). To the best of my knowledge, no breakthrough epidemiological or clinical studies have identified a population of adults as having ADHD who were not previously diagnosed in childhood. Yet it is clear that "adult ADHD" has become a more common and more widely accepted diagnosis in recent years. Dr. Joseph Biederman, a prominent ADHD researcher, claims there are 8 million ADHD adults (*AMA Science News,* 2004). A recent national survey estimated a 4.4 percent prevalence of adult ADHD (Kessler et al., 2006a). A 2004 prescription study reported that 1 percent of the population aged 20–64 now take ADHD drugs, and the number quadrupled from 2000 to 2004 among adults aged 20–44 (Gardiner, 2005). What would bring adults to physicians seeking such a diagnosis and what spurs physicians to treat them? Several social factors appear to have contributed to the diagnostic expansion.

The Prozac Era

The introduction of chlorpromazine in 1955 launched a psychopharmacological revolution in psychiatry (Healy, 1997). Psychoactive medications played a major role in deinstitutionalization, and some (e.g., Valium) became regular parts of physicians' treatment protocols for various life problems, especially anxiety. American psychiatrists preferred drugs that would be useful in office psychiatry rather than medications limited to inpatient populations (Healy, 1997: 70).

In 1987, Prozac (fluoxetine) was introduced as a new type of medication to treat depression. This drug is a selective serotonin reuptake inhibitor that directly affects a different group of neurotransmitters with fewer unpleasant side effects than previous types of antidepressants. This drug quickly became a phenomenon in itself and led to a whole new class of drugs for treating psychiatric and life problems. Peter Kramer's book *Listening to Prozac* (1993) and the subsequent news media coverage (e.g., cover stories in *Newsweek* and *New York* magazines and dozens of television and radio appearances) piqued the public interest in this new drug. Prozac was increasingly depicted as a psychic energizer that could make people feel, in Kramer's terms, "better than well." Prozac was not solely a medication for the seriously disturbed; it could also improve the lives of people with minor psychological difficulties and distresses.

The popularity of Prozac (and a series of related medications) created a social context wherein it was considered acceptable to use medications to treat life's minor problems (cf. Diller, 1996). Just as Prozac was available to people who had redefined their life woes in terms of mild depression, so Ritalin was now available to adults who had not been diagnosed as hyperactive in childhood but who were now redefining their life difficulties as related to "inattention," "impulsivity," and "restlessness." The possibility that adults could "have" ADHD became common in parts of the culture, and many individuals "recognized" that they too had the disorder and sought treatment from physicians. For example, Hallowell and Ratey (1994) recount a case in which a patient demanded Ritalin for his as yet to be officially diagnosed condition. As physicians have come to view ADHD symptoms as not limited to children, they are likely to offer an ADHD diagnosis and a "trial on Ritalin" to adults with certain kinds of life difficulties. The key here, however, is that our culture seems to be moving away from "pharmacological Calvinism" (Klerman cited in Healy, 1997) to the idea that designer drugs might improve the functioning of almost anyone.

Genetics

Genetics is the rising paradigm in medicine, and an increasing number of human problems are being attributed to genetic associations, markers, or causes (Conrad, 1999). Some experts have long believed that there is a genetic component to ADHD and its predecessor, hyperactivity. However, to date, the evidence is only suggestive, even though the claims of inheritance date back at least twenty-five years (Wender, 1971; Cantwell, 1975; Wood et al., 1976). After reviewing extant evidence, researchers noted, "Family, twin, adoption and molecular genetic studies show that it has a substantial genetic component" (Faraone and Beiderman, 1998: 951). Recent research has focused on a genetically induced imbalance of dopamine. Researchers posit a potential link between ADHD and three genes: the D4 dopamine receptor gene, the dopamine transporter gene, and the D2 dopamine receptor gene (Faraone and Beiderman, 1998). The thinking is that people who carry the gene overproduce dopamine, and this overproduction impairs self-control. At least seven genes have been implicated as influencing susceptibility to ADHD (Okie, 2006). Some have suggested that genetic inheritance may account for as much as 80 percent of the likelihood that one has ADHD (Barkley, 1997: 39). Despite the research and much published testimony (e.g., parents reiterating of their ADHD child, "I was just like that when I was his age"), the genetic nature of ADHD is still contested.

However, the greater the medical and public acceptance of a genetic component of ADHD, the more adult ADHD becomes a social reality. If the disorder is genetic, then it is deemed an intrinsic characteristic of people with the gene. This supports the notion that ADHD is a lifelong disorder, and the position that adults could have the disorder even though they were never diagnosed as children.[12]

The Rise of Managed Care

Managed care affects all aspects of medicine, including psychiatry. Health insurance imposes strict limits on the amount of psychotherapy allowed for individual patients. Psychiatrists now must make use of utilization review and participate in medication management, consultation, or administering "carve-out programs" (Domino et al., 1998). Mental health advocates and some researchers argue that under managed care, there is a growing reliance on various forms of prescription therapies to treat all types of psychiatric and life problems (D. Johnson, 1998). A recent study found that managed care may fuel growth in the pharmaceutical industry (Murray and Deardorff, 1998). Undoubtedly, there are now greater incentives for psychiatrists and other physicians to treat all potential mental health problems with medication rather than with some form of "talking therapy" or psychotherapy. Managed care tends to replace psychiatrists with primary care physicians who are less versed in "talking therapies" (Stoudemire, 1996); it thereby increases the potential for relying on medication for treatment. Searight and McLaren (1998) describe a "pragmatic assessment and treatment" that occurs when primary care physicians diagnose and treat ADHD children with pharmaceuticals. In fact, there is some evidence that ADHD children are treated with stimulant medications to the exclusion of "talking therapies" (Wolraich et al., 1990). It is likely that there are similar trends with adult ADHD.

Furthermore, this apparent treatment preference may encourage the expansion of diagnoses of conditions that may be treated with drugs, because these interventions are reimbursable under managed care. Problems that might have been diagnosed differently two decades ago (e.g., adult adjustment reaction) or seen as life dissatisfaction now can be diagnosed and treated as ADHD. While I do not claim that managed care has caused the rise of adult ADHD, it is part of the context that makes ADHD a more likely diagnosis than in the past.

SOME CONSEQUENCES OF THE ADULT ADHD DIAGNOSIS

Three decades ago I outlined some of the ramifications of the medicalization of hyperactive behavior (Conrad, 1975). These ramifications included (1) the problem of expert control, relinquishing authority over problems to experts like physicians; (2) the uses of medical social control, especially drug and surgical treatments; (3) the individualization of social problems; and (4) the depoliticization of deviant behavior, wherein behavior is seen only in terms of its clinical, rather than social, meaning. To these I later added the dislocation of responsibility from the individual to the nether world of biophysiological functioning (Conrad and Schneider, 1992).

Most of these considerations can be applied to adult ADHD as well. The self-initiated and even self-diagnosed nature of most adult ADHD puts a different emphasis on some of these issues (e.g., depoliticization), but it does not neutralize them. With adult ADHD, the shift from personal responsibility and the individualization of life problems may be most critical. Creating a "medical excuse" directs attention away from social forces to biogenic ones and shifts blame from the person to the body. Thus, adult ADHD carries with it some unique consequences, especially because most cases are self-referred adults.

The Medicalization of Underperformance

What is interesting about adult ADHD is that many of those who are given the diagnosis are by some measures successful individuals. Ratey and Hallowell, for example, are both psychiatrists affiliated with a major medical school and authors of a best-selling book, yet they identify themselves as having ADHD. Frank Wolkenberg, who also claimed to have ADHD, was a successful freelance artist. In a widely publicized and controversial article, James Trilling characterized both himself (a professor and author) and his late father, the renowned literary critic Lionel Trilling, as having ADHD (Trilling, 1999). Both lay and professional accounts of adult ADHD commonly provide examples of adults who have achieved success by many conventional social measures (e.g., Hallowell and Ratey, 1994; Leffers, 1997). There are, of course, individuals with limited achievement who are also defined as having ADHD, but the issues remain similar. In fact, Hallowell and Ratey see their audience as "chronic underachievers" whose difficulties are caused not by a lack of self-discipline but by an inborn neurological condition.

For adults, the issue surrounding ADHD is performance, not behavior. As Diller notes, "In broadest terms, moving from childhood to later life for those with ADD involves a shift from problems with behavior to problems with performance. The simple fact of hyperactivity or impulsivity is not the chief concern for teens and adults: rather, it's their disorganization, irresponsibility, procrastination, and inability to complete tasks" (1997: 277).

The adult ADHD diagnosis often stems from a perception of underperformance. This underperformance can be reflected in how tasks are accomplished, continual problematic adaptations, or the level of success achieved. Individuals feel that they could/should be doing better, and they seek help in improving their performance. The ADHD diagnosis provides a medical explanation for their underperformance, allows for the reevaluation of past behavior, and, by shifting responsibility for problems, reduces self-blame. A man who has come to see his ADHD as underlying the chaos in his life said, "I always thought I was stupid" (quoted in Hales and Hales, 1993: 64). Laura, a minister, "always did very well, was always at or near the top of her class through high school, and seminary. . . . But now she told [the psychiatrist that] academics had always been a struggle for her" (Hallowell and Ratey, 1994: 83–84). Another woman reflected, "I had 38 years of thinking I was a bad person. Now I'm rewriting the tapes of who I thought I was to who I really am" (Wallis, 1994: 43).

Beyond an explanation, Ritalin provides a strategy for improving underperformance. Ritalin has been credited with saving marriages, rebuilding faltering careers, and transforming what had been problematic personalities. For example, "Once Sam's ADD was diagnosed, he started on Ritalin at a dosage of 10 mg three times a day, and it worked well in helping him focus and reducing his mood swings" (Hallowell and Ratey, 1994: 111). A 43-year-old woman reports, "I was able to sit down and listen to what my husband had done at work. Shortly after, I was able to sit in bed and read while my husband watched TV" (Wallis, 1994: 49). Some even describe a personal epiphany after first taking Ritalin: "The first day after starting to take the medication, walking down the Brooklyn street on which I then lived, I noticed the sky through the leaves of a tree and stopped to look at it. After a minute it struck me that for the first time in my life I was looking at something with no sensation of having to stop and move on" (Wolkenberg, 1987: 82).

A New Disability

A diagnosis of ADHD puts an individual into the larger category of having a "disability," which can serve as a gateway to potential claims to certain benefits and accommodations. Within this "rights" framework, the diagnosis has been interpreted primarily as a learning disorder (rather than as a psychiatric disorder). While previous research has analyzed the role of ADHD-based claims to rights within children's education (cf. Searight and McLaren, 1998), the expansion of the diagnosis permits the medicalization of adult ADHD to gain further legal validity within the institutions of medicine as well as in employment and adult education.

As ADHD was coming to be identified as a disorder among adults in the early 1990s, individuals began to pursue legal actions to lay claim to rights under legislation such as the Americans with Disabilities Act (ADA) and the Rehabilitation Act of 1973. Although rights are guaranteed under these statutes, they are enforceable only through civil suit. ADHD is not one of the conditions explicitly covered under the ADA, yet advocates have argued that the disorder falls under the umbrella of the law. When ADHD is of sufficient severity to affect an otherwise qualified individual by limiting a major life activity, protections are afforded under the ADA (Latham and Latham, 1995). Individuals with ADHD have filed suits in order to receive reasonable accommodations in education and in the workplace (Jaffe, 1995). For example, a search using the legal database of Lexis-Nexis identified 211 cases in federal labor law between 1980 and 1999 that concern ADHD (many of which include school boards or universities).

Clearly, a diagnosis of adult ADHD carries with it a certain currency in the public sphere. The public is aware of these disability-related issues. In 1993 a key article appeared in the *Wall Street Journal* that outlined workplace and criminal justice issues for those with ADHD. A book on ADD-related disability law was published for advocates in 1992 (Latham and Latham, 1992). Not only are individuals with ADHD the potential beneficiaries of a "medical excuse" for their life problems, but they also may be eligible for specific benefits under the ADA. Individuals who, before diagnosis, would not have seen themselves as having a disability, find themselves reaping the benefits of disability legislation. Under the ADA, individuals with ADHD are entitled to "reasonable accommodations" if their disorder is severe enough to interfere with tasks that they are otherwise qualified to perform. Accommodations could include untimed tests, oral versus written administration of tests or instructions, additional time to complete tasks, structured work assignments with written instructions, extra clerical support, more frequent performance appraisals, checklists for multistage tasks, diminished-capacity arguments in criminal suits, and protection against discrimination (taken from Latham and Latham, 1995; Nadeau 1995a). The 1997 guidelines from the Equal Employment Opportunity Commission (EEOC) led to a list of accommodations for ADHD-diagnosed employees. These accommodations include special office furniture, equipment such as tape recorders and laptops, and "organizational schemes (color coding, buddy systems, alarm clocks, and other 'reminders') designed to keep such employees on track" (Eberstadt, 1999).

ADULT ADHD AND EXPANSION OF A MEDICALIZED CATEGORY

Adult ADHD offers a clear example of how a medicalized category can expand to include a wider range of troubles within its definition. ADHD's expansion was primarily accomplished by refocusing the diagnosis on inattention rather than hyperactivity and stretching the age criteria. This allowed for the inclusion of an entire population of people (and their problems) who were excluded by the original conception of hyperactive children.

The expanded category of adult ADHD has become what Ian Hacking terms "an object of knowledge" with discernable symptoms, putative causes, and particular treatment and care (1995: 96). Adult ADHD is recognized widely as an entity that is real, a "natural category" that only needs proper application. While thirty years ago "adult ADHD" might have been an oxymoron, today it is deemed a discrete disorder that can be claimed and diagnosed.

What is particularly interesting about the adult ADHD case is the role of lay groups in promoting its expansive medicalization. The lay-professional alliance (see also Leffers, 1997), best exemplified by CHADD but also evident in media presentations, suggests an alignment between the claims of patients and professionals. This collaboration contrasts sharply with the case of multiple chemical sensitivity disorder, for which there is a clear-cut disjunction between lay claims-makers and skeptical professionals (Kroll-Smith and Floyd, 1997), and chronic fatigue syndrome, for which individuals may have a difficult time getting their symptoms medically legitimated (L. Cooper, 1997). The lay promotion of adult ADHD and the predominance of self-diagnosis contradict some of the basic premises of the labeling theory of psychiatric diagnosis (Scheff, 1984); this contradiction suggests a fundamental conflict between social control agents and those considered to be deviants. In the case of adult ADHD, the diagnosis is embraced and promoted by the people who receive it. It thus may be a different kind of psychiatric diagnosis from those that sociologists typically study, one that is sought out by the very people to whom it is to be applied. In this case, treatment with medication may be seen as much as an enhancement as a form of social control.

Studies have shown that the interaction of lay and professional claims-makers rather than "medical imperialism" typically underlies the medicalization process. But the case of adult ADHD indicates that popularization may also play a part in diagnostic expansion. Media, including television, popular literature, and the Internet, spread the word quickly about illnesses and treatment. This popularization of symptoms and diagnoses can create new "markets" for disorders and empower previously unidentified individuals to seek treatment as new or expanded medical explanations become available. The widespread popular acceptance of entities as illnesses suggests a "feedback loop" among professionals, claims-makers, media, and the public in terms of the creation, expansion, and application of illness categories. Just as medicalization research has moved from focusing primarily on the claims and activities of physicians to examining the interplay of professional and lay claims-makers, it behooves us to investigate how medical diagnoses penetrate in the public consciousness and become "taken-for-granted as an objective natural entity" in the public sphere (Horwitz, 2002). Such medical diagnostic entities are often accepted without recognizing their history and with an assumption of their universal categorical significance regardless of cultural context. Within an increasingly medically aware public reside individuals who take identified "symptoms" as revealing an underlying disease condition and who, in cases like adult ADHD, may seek to attain their diagnosis of choice.

In 2002, Eli Lilly's drug Strattera (atomoxetine hydrochloride) became the first drug specifically approved and promoted for the treatment of ADHD in adults (see www.strattera.com/1_4_adult_adhd/1_4_adult.jsp). Lilly started a marketing campaign that included television commercials to make the public more aware of adult ADHD. The ads depicted a distracted man forgetting his car keys, arriving late for appointments, and unable to complete work assignments on time, implying that these were symptoms of adult ADHD. By the end of 2004 more than 2 million patients (not all of them adults) were using Strattera, and the FDA voiced some concerns about potential adverse effects (FDA, 2004). More recently, other drugs (e.g., Adderall XR and Focalin) have been approved for adult ADHD. The emergence of adult ADHD and the FDA approval of these medications has more than doubled the pharmaceutical companies' previous pediatric market for these drugs.

In terms of diagnostic expansion, however, the ADHD case is not unique. We can point to other cases in which medicalized categories originally developed and legitimated for one set of problems were extended or reframed to include a broader range of problems. Several examples come to mind. Post-traumatic stress disorder (PTSD) was originally conceived of as a disorder of returning Vietnam war veterans who experienced the aftereffects of brutal combat experience (e.g., with flashbacks, sleep problems, and intense anxiety) (W. Scott, 1990; Young, 1995). In recent years, however, PTSD has been applied to rape and incest survivors, disaster victims, and witnesses to violence. Alcoholism was medicalized in large part because of the efforts of Alcoholics Anonymous (Conrad and Schneider, 1992), but the medicalization has expanded to include adult children of alcoholics, enablers, and especially "codependency" (L. Irvine, 1999). Child abuse, which was originally limited to battering, has expanded to include sexual abuse and neglect and, to a lesser extent, child pornography and exploitation (cf. Best, 1990, 1999). To a degree, it also has spawned the larger domain of domestic violence (including woman battering and elder abuse). In 1972, multiple personality disorder was a rare diagnosis (estimated at less than a dozen cases in fifty years); by 1992, thousands of "multiples" had been diagnosed. This "epidemic" resulted from the diagnostic reconceptualization of multiple personality disorder to "dissociative identity disorder" in DSM-III-R, with less restrictive criteria and an association with child abuse (Hacking, 1995).[13]

Definitional categories are potentially elastic and can be stretched to include more phenomena. This may be particularly true with medicalized categories because of the social advantages of medical definitions (e.g., mitigation of personal blame, medical excuse, health insurance or disability benefits), although fiscal constraints of medicine may set limits on certain applications (Conrad, 2000). While in general the expansion of medical categories may be limited by the carrying capacity of the medical profession and the health insurance industry (cf. Hilgartner and Bosk, 1988), it appears that with active claims-makers, committed stakeholders, and receptive potential clients, diagnostic expansion can occur readily and with minimal opposition. Similar to domain expansion, diagnostic expansion begins with established disorders and moves toward more problematic claims. One legitimated medical category can beget others.

It is interesting to consider whether a parallel process of diagnostic contraction may take place. Some have suggested that this narrowing has occurred for serious mental illness. With the increased reliance on primary care providers in managed care, for example, some research has suggested an underrecognition of some serious mental disorders (Stoudemire, 1996). Others have noted that the "medical necessity" standard has altered, not only for treatment but in diagnosis (Ford, 1998). It stands to reason that in the age of managed care, shrinkage of the medical domain is a likely outcome. Yet, as noted in the adult ADHD example, managed care may have paradoxically played a role in the emergence of this new category. Whatever the ultimate outcome of problem definitions, the flexibility of certain medical diagnoses allows for expansion and thus the increase of medicalization in our society.

CHAPTER FOUR

Enhancement

Human Growth Hormone and the
Temptations of Biomedical Enhancement

This chapter uses the case of human growth hormone (hGH) to examine the social nature of biomedical enhancements. The pharmaceutical industry developed synthetic hGH in 1985, and it was approved by the Food and Drug Administration for specific uses, particularly the treatment of growth hormone deficiency. However, it has also been promoted for several "off-label" (i.e., non-FDA-approved) uses, most of which can be deemed enhancements. Drugs approved for one treatment pave the way for use as enhancements for other problems. Claims have been made for hGH as a treatment for idiopathic shortness, as an antiaging agent, and to improve athletic performance. Biomedical enhancements use medical means to augment the body or performance and are thus forms of medicalization. Using the hGH case, we can see how enhancements can expand the purview of medicalization in society.

It is likely that humans have sought enhancements for themselves or their children for as long as they have recognized that improvements in individuals are a possibility. These might have included strategies, techniques, or potions to make humans stronger, smarter, faster, live longer, or live with keener senses. In contemporary society, parents seek to enhance their children's life chances by providing music lessons, tutoring, private-school education, after-school programs, summer camps, and the like. Adults may endeavor to enhance themselves with supplements, exercise workouts, special courses, and diverse cultural experiences. There is no shortage of methods of self-improvement (Schur, 1976), many of which could be called enhancements.

One particular genre of self-improvement in modern society is "biomedical enhancements." These include drugs, surgery, and other medical interventions aimed at improving one's mind, body, or performance. Cosmetic surgery, including liposuction, face lifts, breast augmentation, and "nose jobs" (Sullivan, 2001), has become a common biomedical road to bodily improvement. Performance-enhancing drugs such as steroids, hormones, and stimulant medications, often used by competitive athletes, have caused controversy. More recently, Peter Kramer (1993) conceptualized certain drugs like Prozac as having the potential qualities of "cosmetic psychopharmacology," making individuals "better than well."

There has been considerable social concern about the potential of genetic engineering as a new and particularly powerful form of biomedical enhancement. While genetic enhancements are yet to be developed, many experts believe that they are likely to be available in some form in the not so distant future (Silver, 1997; Buchanan et al., 2000). The potential of genetics has been the focus of the current debate on enhancement. Maxwell Mehlman defined genetic intervention as an enhancement when (1) it is undertaken for the purposes of improving a characteristic or capability that, but for the enhancement, would lie within what is generally accepted as a normal range for humans; or when (2) it installs a characteristic or capability that is not normally present in human beings (2000: 523). The first type of enhancement would include greater cognitive abilities, improved physical performance, or augmented body size or function. The second might include the ability to see clearly at night, glow in the dark, or grow wings (cf. Slater, 2001). For now, the latter types of enhancement are mostly science fictions, but the possibilities remain.

What constitutes a biomedical enhancement is not always clear. Eric Juengst, a bioethicist, suggests that "the term enhancement is usually used in bioethics to characterize interventions designed to improve human form or functioning beyond what is necessary to sustain or restore human health" (1998: 29). From a sociological point of view, however, it is not necessarily obvious what is "human form or functioning beyond . . . human health" because, as social constructionists and others have pointed out, the definition of health is socially situated, is flexible, and may ultimately be a mirage (Dubos, 1959). Because there is no universally accepted definition of health, it would be difficult to imagine a consensus on what going beyond health to enhancement might be. The line between the two is movable and the boundaries are likely to be heavily contested.

Some analysts believe we can draw a hard line between treatments and enhancements. Treatments are for real medical diseases, while enhancements are for bodily or performance improvements. As Norman Daniels (1994) states, "Characterizing medical need implies a contrast between medical services to treat disease (or disability) conditions and uses that merely enhance human performance or appearance" (quoted in Parens, 1998: 4). This view assumes that agreement exists about what a disease is and that we can separate disease-driven treatments from interventions for people without a recognizable malady. Biomedical interventions without a malady would probably be seen as "merely" an enhancement. But what constitutes a medical need is not self-evident and may differ by society and shift over time. New diseases or disorders may be defined (as diagnoses) in order to legitimate medical treatments or interventions (Conrad, 1992, 2000). Thus, the line between what is deemed a necessary treatment and what is an enhancement can be blurred and can shift as definitions of disease change. If, for example, scientists developed a drug that could enhance memory, we might soon see a growth of diagnoses of "memory deficit disorder." Would this be a treatment or an enhancement? The boundaries of disease and enhancement are likely to be severely contested, especially by those who want interventions legitimated as therapies for medical problems.

The context of an intervention may determine not only if an intervention is an enhancement but also whether it is deemed acceptable or illicit. To borrow an example from David Frankford, it would be obligatory for physicians to prescribe Cognex for memory loss resulting from Alzheimer disease; it would be legitimate for students to take it to improve their college admissions test scores; but it would be illegal for international chess players to take it to strengthen their match play (1998: 71). In the first instance, Cognex intervention could be deemed a necessary medical treatment, and in the second, a permitted means of betterment, while in the third it would be deemed an illegitimate performance enhancement. As Frankford notes, treatment for "memory 'loss' in Alzheimer's 'restores' a 'natural' function, founded in biological processes . . . [while] using Cognex to play chess better creates 'additional' memory, akin to that of a computer, something 'artificial' founded in technology not biology" (p. 72). The natural/artificial dichotomy is unlikely to be the core of the issue here. Rather, in the Alzheimer's case, the drug intervention is deemed a "repair" while in the chess case it provides an "augmentation" that creates an unfair advantage. While Cognex might also provide an advantage in the college admissions test case, it could be considered legitimate until proved otherwise. In all three cases, memory has been improved by taking the drug, but they are different kinds of enhancements. Enhancements are additive to the condition—frequently, but not always, taking the body or performance to where it either has never been or wishes to return.

Biomedical enhancements are interventions that are usually provided in a medical context through surgery, pharmacology, or genetic intervention. Some biomedical enhancements are available without medical supervision; these include herbal remedies, supplements, and many performance-enhancing drugs. Medical personnel are often but not always involved. Biomedical enhancements may get the most publicity or create the greatest concerns, but they are by no means the only kinds of enhancements. Socially based enhancements, such as after-school programs, tutoring, music lessons, or special courses, are common. Mental techniques like meditation, mind control, and cognitive memory improvement aids might also be enhancements. It is not always clear where the line between "enrichment" and "enhancement" lies: are music lessons enrichment while test tutoring is enhancement? Is one considered enrichment because it broadens the child's experience and the other enhancement because the goal is to improve the test score? In a real sense, these distinctions are definitional and contextual.

This chapter examines the development of synthetic human growth hormone and its subsequent off-label uses for biomedical enhancement, specifically with idiopathic short stature, aging, and athletic performance. Because of its myriad uses, hGH is a particularly good example to consider as a means to investigate types of biomedical enhancement and the social dilemmas associated with them. This chapter focuses on developments in the United States, but the issues are broadly applicable.

THE EMERGENCE OF HUMAN GROWTH HORMONE
The Development of Synthetic hGH

Children who experience what is considered normal growth secrete enough human growth hormone from their own pituitary gland to stimulate bodily growth from conception through puberty. Before 1985, individuals who had a deficiency in natural hGH were treated with hGH extracted from the pituitary glands of cadavers. The treatment of children diagnosed with growth hormone deficiency was very expensive. Furthermore, because the growth hormone was in such low supply, it was given only to hGH-deficient young children in the lowest three percentiles in height for their age and sex (*Newsweek*, 1985: 70). Even so, the supply could not meet the demand; the number of hGH-deficient children in the United States was estimated by some to be 10,000 (Erickson, 1990: 164) and by others to be as high as 15,000 to 20,000 (Werth, 1991; Patlak, 1992: 31). There was a constant shortage of cadaver-extracted hGH.

By 1985, considerable health risks were becoming apparent. Four people who had received the cadaver-extracted hormone as children later died from Creutzfeldt-Jakob disease, a fatal degeneration of the brain with severe neurological signs and symptoms. Death occurs over the course of a year. Scientists originally believed that the cause of these Creutzfeldt-Jakob cases was a virus in the cadaver-extracted hormone. That same year (1985), the National Institutes of Health removed this hormone from the market.

Fortunately for patients who required hGH, the biotechnology company Genentech had already developed a synthetic version of human growth hormone. The synthetic hGH, called Protropin, had been in development for almost a decade (*Newsweek*, 1985: 70) and received FDA approval shortly after the cadaver extract was removed from the market. Scientists at Genentech first used recombinant DNA technology to synthesize the genetic blueprint of hGH. This process was identified as a safe alternative to the cadaver-extracted hGH. The recombinant substance could be produced in "potentially unlimited quantities" (Lantos et al., 1989: 1020), and physicians credited the new technology with ending the market shortage of the hormone (Glasbrenner, 1986). Finally, the product was priced at the relatively affordable amount of approximately $8,000 per year of treatment (Abramson, 1985: 70), though more recent estimates are $15,000–20,000 annually (Lantos et al., 1989: 1020; Werth, 1991).

These three factors (the product's safety, increased quantity, and low cost) made the pharmaceutical version attractive to existing and potential patients. Genentech quickly supplied the needs of the existing market and claimed 75 percent of the U.S. market for a total of $200 million (Werth, 1991: 28). Claims began to surface that the biotech manufacturer was establishing other distribution outlets that involved off-label uses of Protropin. The synthetic hGH is a schedule III drug and therefore must be distributed through prescription by a licensed physician, according to USC21 §333(e). Yet the FDA had approved the hormone only for use in treating the medical problem of hypopituitary dwarfism (or growth hormone deficiency) and chronic renal failure (Bercu, 1996).

The diagnostic criteria for assessing growth hormone deficiency are stringent but have been contested. Criteria include (1) height of more than three standard deviations below the mean for the child's age, (2) abnormal growth velocity (less than the twenty-fifth percentile for bone age), and (3) GH provocative testing results with peak GH of less than 10 μg/L in a polyclonal radioimmunoassay (Bercu, 1996). It is this latter criterion that has produced the most controversy (Lantos et al., 1989; Bercu, 1996). For example, peak GH levels between 7 and 10 are considered a "gray zone," and different methods of assessing GH levels produce varying results (Lantos et al., 1989). Nonetheless, while individual cases might be disputed, the medical profession has established guidelines to distinguish between growth hormone deficiency and what has been called idiopathic short stature (normal growth hormone levels in children who are short).

Seeking Off-Label Uses

While physicians, in practice, have the autonomy and authority to prescribe off label,[1] manufacturers cannot legally market their products for off-label uses. In the case of synthetic human growth hormone, Genentech and other pharmaceutical companies could not legally market the drug for anything but its FDA-approved conditions, which had diagnostic criteria established by the medical profession.

As time went on, physicians, patients, and drug companies all sought other medical uses for hGH. By 1990, researchers and leading drug companies were investigating the possibility of administering hGH to children with idiopathic short stature. A national survey of 534 pediatric endocrinologists documented that approximately 94 percent of them had prescribed hGH for non-growth-hormone-deficient children within the previous five years (Cutler et al., 1996: 532). Furthermore, Genentech, and to some extent Eli Lilly (another manufacturer of hGH), worked closely with the Human Growth Foundation, a nonprofit advocacy group that supported "short children" (Werth, 1991)—a more general term encompassing both hypopituitary dwarfism and idiopathic short stature. Genentech also supported research by pediatric endocrinologists and began its own longitudinal research on "healthy" children who were not hormone deficient. These activities further blurred the boundaries demarcating "legitimate" and "off-label" use of hGH.

Other off-label uses arose. For example, physicians would prescribe the drug to fight "wasting" in AIDS patients, because hGH was believed to increase weight gain and guard against muscle loss (Erickson, 1990; Hilchey, 1994). Genentech reported that the hormone was helping "severely burned children heal faster," and others said it helped cancer patients maintain weight during chemotherapy treatment (Erickson, 1990). Some physicians prescribed the hormone as treatment for chronic renal insufficiency as well as for osteoporosis, obesity, and trauma (Erickson, 1990; Bradley and Sodeman, 1990). Other physicians and patients believed hGH had antiaging properties (Cowley, 1996; Rae, 1996; Stabinger, 1999).

Federal Investigations

In 1994 several federal agencies began a series of investigations targeting Eli Lilly and Genentech for overpromoting their growth hormone products—that is, marketing them for nonapproved uses (R. Weiss, 1993; Mintz, 1995; Auerbach, 1996; Amoroso, 1999).[2] Initial interest was stimulated by a *New York Times* article that appeared in June 1991 (Werth, 1991), prompting an FDA inspection in 1992.

Beginning in 1994 and lasting through 1995, the Food and Drug Administration and the Federal Bureau of Investigation interviewed people connected with Genentech's marketing effort, including employees of Caremark, the distributor of Protropin. The FDA believed that Genentech sales of Protropin for unapproved uses grossed $20 million (Nordenberg, 1999: 33), and in 1995 the FDA requested that Genentech turn over all company documents relating to the promotion and marketing of Protropin.

Meanwhile, the House Committee on Small Business (Subcommittee on Regulation, Business Opportunities, and Technology), chaired by Representative Ron Wyden, had called for a series of congressional hearings to investigate charges of off-label promotion by the biotech manufacturers. Among the allegations investigated were charges that "doctors were receiving cash payoffs, sometimes disguised as 'research grants,' to prescribe hormone drugs to patients even when they lacked obvious clinical diagnosis of hormone deficiency" (Wyden, 1994).

A range of testimony was heard on October 12, 1994, from government administrators, physicians, advocates, and parents. A written statement prepared by Genentech outlined its "comprehensive clinical research program" to evaluate the safe uses of Protropin and claimed it had developed a "tightly controlled distribution system" ensuring that its "hGH products were available only to patients who medically need them" (Genentech, 1994).

Mark W. Parker, M.D., a practicing pediatric endocrinologist from North Carolina who had been asked to testify by Rep. Wyden, described his procedure for diagnosing and treating hormone-deficient short stature. He essentially supported Genentech's claims of no off-label use: "I have never prescribed growth hormone where it was not medically indicated. . . . Growth hormone is assuredly not appropriate for treatment for most short children. However, in the growth hormone deficient child, such therapy was not only indicated but potentially life changing" (Parker, 1994).

Fran Price, from the Human Growth Foundation (HGF, a nonprofit agency that receives some funding from Genentech and participates in school height screening programs), submitted testimony; the HGF had not been invited to testify to the panel. She pointed out that experts see growth as an important indicator of a child's overall health and support in-school screenings to reach "children who may not otherwise have access to preventive care": "Our goal regarding the treatment of growth disorders is not to make all children tall, but rather, to help all children remain as healthy and grow as normally as possible" (Price, 1994).

Not all the testimony was so positive. Stanley Dobrin, whose two sons had been treated for growth-hormone-deficient disorders between 1982 and 1993, stated that "growth hormone is easy to promote. There is no resistance, no questioning, when you, as a parent, are dealing with your child's welfare. Growth hormone therapy can easily be exploited by any doctor who may be more interested in how much money he or she can make than the true medical needs of the children he or she is treating" (Dobrin, 1994).

Although the congressional investigation of Eli Lilly and Genentech was extensive, no federal charges were brought (e.g., R. Weiss, 1993; Auerbach, 1996). The hearings could not substantiate claims that Genentech had used illegal means to promote the use of Protropin. Yet as a result of the continuing investigations by the FBI and the FDA, Genentech was subject to criminal prosecution in 1999 and settled under a plea agreement before judgment was reached on the case. For its part, the FDA alleged and documented that by the end of 1985, Genentech had "begun marketing Protropin for use in the treatment of medical conditions for which it did not have FDA approval" (Nordenberg, 1999: 33). From 1985 to 1994, Genentech marketed Protropin to a variety of medical practitioners (doctors, hospitals, and others) for treating unapproved conditions, including idiopathic short stature. Genentech paid $50 million in settlement, including a $20 million penalty to reimburse Medicaid and CHAMPUS (Nordenberg, 1999).

FDA restrictions on manufacturers have recently been eased, broadening the information they may provide to physicians about off-label uses of their products (Stapleton, 1999). These restrictions were loosened by the Food and Drug Administration Modernization Act, endorsed by the AMA, which was passed in 1997 and put into effect the following year. Drug manufacturers could now disseminate off-label information that had been published in peer-reviewed scientific journals, if (1) the article was "balanced,"(2) the use was clearly marked as off-label, and (3) the company had the necessary trials in place to eventually ask for supplemental approval from the FDA.

HGH AND HUMAN ENHANCEMENT

The relative ease with which manufacturers may promote and physicians may prescribe hGH for off-label treatment has increased the range of possible uses. At least two medically sanctioned uses have dominated the literature: as a treatment for idiopathic short stature and as an antiaging therapy. A third use, to enhance athletic performance, though not medically sanctioned, is reportedly common. In a sense, hGH can be seen as a case study in the potentials and temptations of human biomedical enhancement.

Idiopathic Short Stature

Virtually all human populations contain a range of heights. One could argue that any height not produced by disease or dysfunction is just one point on the potential human height scale. But because height is imbued with certain social meanings and in some cases (e.g., extreme shortness) can become stigmatized, not all heights are considered equal.

Throughout the twentieth century, Americans got taller. Only 10.4 percent of men born between 1906 and 1915 were over 6 feet tall, while 31.8 percent of those born a half-century later (1956–62) were over 6 feet. The average increase in height can be seen on the short end of the spectrum as well: 29.4 percent of the men born in the earlier period were less than 5 feet 7 inches, while only 8.2 percent born in the more recent period were that short. Women born between 1956 and 1962 were five times more likely to be over 5 feet 5 inches tall than women born between 1906 and 1915 (cited in Konner, 1999). Changes in height also occurred elsewhere. In Japan, today's children are 3 to 5 inches taller than their grandparents (Samaras, 1995). These increases in height are usually attributed to better nutrition and rising standards of living.[3]

When populations get taller, there are changes in height across the spectrum, but extremely short (or tall) individuals remain. In Western society, at least, shortness, and especially extreme shortness, is often devalued and can have consequences, especially for males. One might see this as a form of "heightism," whereby short people become stigmatized. Cultural stereotypes reflect attitudes toward stature. Stature seems to be more consequential for men, although it may be significant for women as well (Keyes, 1980). Attractive men are "tall, dark, and handsome," while short stature is perceived as immature and childlike. Words in our language reflect our attitudes toward shortness: "shrimp," "small fry," "squirt," "half-pint." Randy Newman's ironic song seemed to denigrate short people with the chorus, "Short people got no reason to live." Figures of speech involving shortness are often negative: "getting the short end of the stick," "coming up short." We "look down" with contempt and "look up" with respect. A lack of height can have more direct effects as well: "Short stature is clearly associated with a perception that such men are immature and weak. Being a very short male is the type of characteristic that is related to a higher risk of maltreatment by family members and peers" (Martel and Biller, 1987: 25).

It has been reported that short children are teased or babied because of their stature (Sandberg, 1999), but the consequences are unclear. A review of extant studies noted that while between one-half and three-quarters of short children are treated as younger than their actual age and teased for their short stature, researchers found no signs of psychosocial maladjustment, and the individuals' quality of life was generally good (Kelnar et al., 1999). Other studies have questioned whether shortness has more than a minimally detectable impact on children (Hall, 2005).

Some evidence suggests that there are social advantages to tallness, although there is no conclusive evidence about the disadvantages of shortness. Generally, "tall people are more likely to be hired for a given job and to have higher salaries in similar jobs" (Diekema, 1990: 111; cf. Bowles et al., 2001; *Economist*, 2002). Irene Frieze and her colleagues (1990) estimated that taller men earned approximately $600 more annually for each inch of height compared with their equally qualified but shorter co-workers. One study found that people holding senior posts in professions were significantly taller than those in junior positions (Schumacher, 1982). Most twentieth-century presidential elections have gone to the taller candidate; since 1952 (the dawn of the TV era), the shorter candidate has won only three times, including 2004 (Diekema, 1990; Mathews, 1999).

There are data to suggest that short men are viewed as less attractive than tall men (Martel and Biller, 1987: 25). There seems to be an assumption regarding individuals' competence based on appearance, with shorter individuals probably subject to some disadvantage. This may affect how people see themselves. One study found that tall men felt more comfortable than short men in a variety of situations (Voss, 1999: 7); overall "the adult studies would seem to indicate that stature and social and economic success may be linked" (p. 9).

Whatever the real or imagined disadvantages of shortness, many parents have anxieties about their children's height. As Leslie Martel and Henry Biller note, "Even if other medical handicaps are not involved, parents generally have a difficult time accepting a diagnosis that their child will remain shorter than average" (1987: 97). Physicians have become good at predicting adult height in children, and such diagnoses may trigger parents' concern. After 1986, when the supply of hGH became more plentiful, parents for the first time could consider interventions that would influence the height of their children.

As noted earlier, short stature is defined by being in the lowest three percentiles for age and sex, which is roughly two standard deviations from the mean; for adult males it is 64.5 inches or less, for adult females it is 59.5 inches (NHANES, 2000). It is estimated that 1.8 million children in the United States and a similar number in Europe can be characterized as being of significantly short stature. Only 20 percent of these are referred to pediatric endocrinologists, and only 5 percent of these are growth-hormone-deficient (Hintz, 1996). The vast majority of short children, therefore, have idiopathic short stature (ISS), defined as "a heterogeneous state that encompasses individuals with short stature, including those with FSS (familial short stature), for which there is no recognized cause" (Kelnar et al., 1999: 151). The causes may well be familial (short parents), genetic, or nutritional, but ISS can be seen as "normal shortness" as opposed to a more specific "deficiency shortness."

Parents typically want to enhance their child's life chances, to give him or her an advantage in life. One manner of doing this would be to treat the ISS child with hGH to increase his or her height. One estimate suggests that at least 13,000 children in the United States with ISS were treated with hGH in 1994.[4] Research on hGH treatment of children with ISS has been equivocal. In general, treatment of ISS children increases the rate of growth in the short run, but the final adult height studies have been inconsistent. It is debatable how much treatment can increase growth from predicted height (see, e.g., Hintz, 1996). One major multicenter study, sponsored by Genentech, reported that of the 80 children who reached final height, the mean gain from predicted height was 5.9 cm (2.3 inches) in girls and 5.0 cm (2 inches) in boys (Hintz et al., 1999). A Dutch study reported a gain of 2.4–4.8 cm (approximately 1–2 inches), where more than half the subjects gained 2 inches or more to final adult height (cited in Kelnar et al., 1999). The height gains are modest; hGH will not transform a short person into a tall one, but only into a less short one. The treatment costs about $20,000 a year and must be continued for three to six years. At an average cost of $100,000 for an average height gain of 2 inches, the cost of height enhancement is roughly $50,000 an inch. Parents must pay for this treatment themselves.

In July 2003 the FDA approved the use of Humatrope, an Eli Lilly version of hGH, to treat the shortest 1.2 percent of children with ISS. This was the first official approval of a drug to treat short children who did not have a growth hormone deficiency. As part of the approval, Lilly agreed not to advertise directly to consumers. The company estimates that 400,000 children could fit this new criterion, although only an expected 10 percent would get treatment (M. Kaufman, 2003). Eli Lilly has distributed its own rendition of the Centers for Disease Control growth chart, with a bright red line at the 1.2 percent mark, hoping to sensitize doctors to the FDA cutoff point and make hGH treatment an option to consider. This decision significantly expands the medical jurisdiction over shortness and increases the possibilities for biomedical enhancement. In the first full year after the approval for expanded use, Pfizer's sales of Genotropin went up 53 percent over the previous year, and Eli Lilly saw a 16 percent increase in the sale of Humatrope (Hall, 2005).

C. J. H. Kelnar and colleagues reported that "the quality of life of adults with ISS is normal both in those treated with hGH during childhood and in those not referred for treatment, although the majority of parents wished to be taller and reported one or more negative effects related to height" (1999: 156) They concluded that there is "no strong evidence hGH therapy improves psychological adaptation of children with ISS" (p. 157). While hGH may add a couple of inches of height, it is not clear whether this has any impact on the social and psychological consequences of short stature.

Those parents who seek treatment for their ISS children may be a self-selected group. One study (Busschbach et al., 1999) compared ISS children who sought treatment for short stature with a group of ISS children who did not ("normal shorts"). The normal shorts perceived much less stigma and problems related to their stature than did their counterparts, and a major difference was the attitude of the parents. Parents who did not find shortness problematic did not seek treatment for their children, and those children enjoyed a much more positive attitude. The authors conclude that short stature is not necessarily a burden. Perhaps the parents and children who present with ISS to endocrinologists have problems that they attribute to shortness but are not necessarily related to it (p. 34). David Sandberg concluded, "It appears that psychosocial stressors associated with SS [short stature] are likely contributing to [the] variability in social competencies and behavior problems that fall within the normal range" (1999: 22). Parents who seek treatment for ISS may be showing complicity with "heightism" and passing this message on to their children. They may thus inadvertently reinforce the stigma of shortness by providing treatment for it, focusing on body size instead of viewing the whole child.

In sum, there is some evidence that short stature is stigmatized in our society and that hGH can enhance a child's adult height by a couple of inches, but it is unclear whether this enhancement will have any effect on the individual's social and psychological functioning. As one doctor put it, "Short stature became a disease when unlimited amounts of growth hormone became available" (quoted in Hall, 2005).

hGH as an Antiaging Agent

Human growth hormone has been hailed as an enhancement that can forestall and even reverse the aging process. Some advocates claim that the hormone can restore the body's performance capacity to its pinnacle, perhaps even to a condition better than it ever was.

In 1990 Dr. Daniel Rudman and colleagues at the Medical College of Wisconsin in Milwaukee published what would become a widely cited report in the *New England Journal of Medicine* (Rudman et al., 1990). They had used hGH experimentally to treat bodily deterioration among a small sample (N = 21) of healthy elderly men, aged 61–81, with low levels of hGH. Rudman's theory was that what he called "growth hormone menopause" (Foreman, 1992) left aging adults with little or no growth hormone, resulting in decreased muscle mass and increased fatty tissue. The proposed remedy was to replenish the lost hGH to restore body composition. In the experiment, after six months of daily hGH injections, those subjects treated with hGH saw their lean body mass increase by 9 percent, their fat decrease by 14 percent, their muscle mass increase, and their skin become less opaque and fragile. Investigators said that the building up of muscle and the reduction in fat were "equivalent in magnitude to the changes incurred during 10 to 20 years of aging" (Rudman et al., 1990: 5).

The antiaging properties of hGH struck a nerve with a certain segment of medical practitioners. Antiaging (now sometimes referred to as "age management") medicine, has become a specialty for a sizable number of health care practitioners, especially practitioners of alternative or complementary medicine. While not endorsed by the American Medical Association, the American Academy of Anti-Aging Medicine (A4M), for example, has provided institutional support for antiaging claims. One of its mottoes is, "Aging is not inevitable!" According to the organization's website (www.worldhealth.net), A4M is a "registered 501(c)3 nonprofit organization that is the sole medical society dedicated to the advancement of therapeutics related to the science of longevity medicine." Its membership includes over ten thousand physicians, health practitioners, and scientists in sixty countries. Many of its activities are designed to increase both the credibility of antiaging therapies and the professional status of its practitioners. The organization offers certification to physicians and other health care practitioners. In addition, A4M offers continuing-education courses for physicians and surgeons, publishes textbooks on antiaging medicine, and sponsors educational features on cable television.

Since the initial Rudman report, however, many mainstream medical researchers have been concerned about the study's scientific limitations and the potential adverse effects of administering hGH. Letters to the editor in subsequent issues of the *New England Journal of Medicine* urged readers to interpret the Rudman study with caution, if not skepticism. Some academic researchers criticized Rudman's findings and questioned the fundamental biological theory underlying the use of hGH to "treat" aging. They concluded that the extent to which age-related changes in growth hormone contribute to changes in bodily composition remains unknown (Corpas et al., 1993). Others (e.g., Taaffe et al., 1994) were unable to replicate Rudman's findings: although lean body mass could be increased and fat decreased in another small sample (N = 18) of healthy elderly men undergoing strength training, supplementation with hGH did not change body weight or increase strength. The benefits of hGH treatment therefore remained questionable.

Four years after a second Rudman study (Rudman et al., 1991), researchers at the University of California at San Francisco and the Veterans' Affairs Medical Center (Papadakis et al., 1996) concluded that hGH not only was an ineffective treatment but also had distinctly unpleasant, if not harmful, side effects. Unlike Rudman's subjects, the 52 elderly male subjects (over age 69) chosen for Papadakis's study were not told the details of their treatment. Although Papadakis and colleagues confirmed some of Rudman's findings, such as an increase in body mass and decrease in fat, other findings were more equivocal. For example, body weight did not change. Furthermore, there were no improvements in functioning (such as in muscle strength, endurance, or mental acuity). Finally, side effects included joint pain, stiff hands, and swelling in the ankles and lower extremities. The study, published in the *Annals of Internal Medicine,* was picked up by the popular media (e.g., *New York Times,* 1996; Saltus, 1996; Butler et al., 2000).

Human growth hormone had begun to capture the media's imagination. The Rudman studies were widely reported in leading newspapers and popular magazines (e.g., Angier, 1990; *New York Times,* 1990; Saltus, 1990; Foreman, 1992). While the researchers had extrapolated the results of their study and claimed that the treatment restored ten to twenty years of aging effects, the claims bandied about in public discourse were more far-reaching, with some likening the hormone to the "fountain of youth" (Saltus, 1990). Some reporters claimed that the treatment could "significantly reverse many effects of aging" (Angier, 1990). Although Rudman himself would try to contain these claims by noting the complexities of the aging process and declaring that the hormone was "not a fountain of youth" (Angier, 1990), these belated cautions went largely unheeded. Similarly, warnings about the risks of using hGH, listed in an editorial published along with the research article (Vance, 1990), did not make mainstream news.

Several institutions emerged to treat aging with hGH, as well as with other medications. One of the first treatment centers was El Dorado Rejuvenation and Longevity Institute, founded near Cancun, Mexico, outside the regulatory jurisdiction of the FDA. Its promotional material described the facility as a "comprehensive medical research and spa resort . . . [which] offers a proven restorative plan that effectively turns back the clock 10 to 20 years" (Lindenman, 1993). During a two-day stay costing $4,600, the guest is taught to self-inject hGH. A three-month supply of the hormone is then shipped to the individual back in the United States. Subsequent refills of the hormone can be obtained through a mail-order arrangement at the institute. Other treatment centers emerged and have benefited from increased exposure on the Internet.

Advocates of antiaging have used educational and distribution outlets on the Internet to spread claims about hGH and other antiaging enhancements (cf. Vincent, 2006). Some websites, such as www.hormoneshop.com, www.vital-solutions.com, and www.antiaging.com, sell antiaging products (including supplements) and educational materials. The supplements offered do not include the synthetic hGH that is manufactured by drug companies such as Genentech and Eli Lilly. Rather, they are variations on these prescription drugs (to bypass the laws controlling prescription drugs) and include such things as homeopathic or natural hGH. Other websites advertise treatment centers that have physicians on staff and can therefore offer hGH treatment as well as other types of enhancements. The Age Reversal Centres, Inc., bills itself as a "fountain of youth," as does the Longevity Center for South Florida. The latter proclaims expertise in "interventional endocrinology," quasi-scientific jargon that frames the center's claims to improve quality of life.

Despite concerns about medical risks and lack of efficacy, the distribution of hGH via websites and antiaging clinics has become a huge industry, with U.S. sales exceeding $700 million in 2004 and worldwide sales estimated at $1.5 billion to $2 billion, with an estimated 30 percent of hGH prescriptions going for antiaging and athletic enhancement (Foreman, 2005; Perls et al., 2005).

hGH and the Enhancement of Athletic Performance

Competitive athletes by nature want to maximize their performances. They may use special training regimens, new techniques, diet and exercise, innovative equipment, or countless other ways to improve performances. In Western sports there seems to be a great concern with distinguishing "between natural and unnatural, the nutrient and the stimulant, the regenerative and the performance enhancing" for improving athletic outcomes, with performance-enhancing drugs being deemed unnatural and often illegal (Hoberman, 1992: 27; 2005: 179–213). Drugs are considered to boost performances "artificially" and to create an uneven playing field. They are seen by many as a danger to the ethos of sport (Hoberman, 1992, 1995, 2005). For example, the Olympic Movement Anti-Doping Code was adopted in 1999, banning certain existing substances as well as those yet to be discovered (usolympicteam.com, 2005). Numerous classes of substances are banned, including hGH, because they "contravene the fundamental principles of Olympianism and sports and medical ethics" (IOC, 2000: article 1).

Athletes have long sought substances that could improve their performances. Ergogenic, or performance-enhancing, aids have a long history. "Olympic athletes in ancient Greece are believed to have used herbs and mushrooms to improve athletic performance," and nineteenth-century French athletes drank *vin mariani*, a mixture of coca leaves and wine that was alleged to reduce the fatigue and hunger associated with prolonged exercise (Wagner, 1989: 2059). Beginning in the 1950s, steroids became the ergogenic drug of choice for athletes, especially those involved in strength and speed sports. These drugs can increase size, strength, and stamina, and although they can have disturbing side effects, the use (and abuse) of these drugs is often difficult to detect. By the mid-1960s so many athletes were using anabolic steroids that the International Olympic Committee (IOC) instituted drug testing in 1968, finally banning steroid use by athletes in 1975. A major scandal occurred during the 1976 Olympics, when the East German swimmers showed great improvement in speed and were subsequently found to have been given steroids as "supplements" to their rigorous training (Curry and Salerno, 1999). By the 1990s, more effective drug testing and a growing awareness of the noxious side effects had reduced the appeal of steroid enhancement.

While many drugs create a bodily risk, it is worth noting that athletes train for performance, not health, so the risk benefit ratio of performance-enhancing drugs is often weighted in favor of taking the drugs. "In a survey of 100 top runners, each was asked if he could take a pill that would allow him to be Olympic champion but kill him in a year, over half the runners said they would take the pill" (Samaras, 1995: 29). Many athletes consider drugs a natural part of training, a necessary evil for success (Wagner, 1989: 2060). In some sports, like power-lifting and football, athletes may feel compelled to use ergogenic drugs because they believe all their competitors do.

Soon after the development of hGH in 1985, the athletic underground began to consider hGH as a drug with great ergogenic potential. While no scientific articles extolling the performance-enhancing qualities of hGH were published, some doctors and athletes began to experiment with using hGH for performance enhancement. Like steroids a decade earlier, the claims remained clandestine and more pragmatic than scientific. Human growth hormone was moderate in cost and relatively easy to obtain, either from willing doctors or on the black market. Athletes and their trainers were interested in hGH for its growth-promoting action on skeletal tissue: "It caused a significant percentage increase in fat free weight and a decrease in fat without a significant retention of extracellular fluid" (Kicman and Cowan, 1992: 504). Some believed that it was "more potent than anabolic steroids or could be used in conjunction with steroids to increase muscular size and strength" (p. 504). Furthermore, hGH is a nonsteroidal anabolic agent that can evade drug tests. Currently there is no reliable method of detection, in part because it is a substance found naturally in the body and because it has a low concentration in urine and is thus nearly undetectable in urine tests. Its concentration is one hundred times higher in the blood, but the International Olympic Committee did not permit blood testing until 2000 (Zorpette, 2000). Despite the lack of a reliable test, in 1989 the IOC banned hGH as part of a new doping class of "peptide hormones and analogues" (Kicman and Cowan, 1992).

There was a great deal of excitement in the athletic world about hGH when it was first introduced. For many athletes it became the new drug of choice (Saugy et al., 1996), with some athletes calling the 1996 Olympics the "hGH games" (Zorpette, 2000). But a few years later, reports about its ergogenic properties were more equivocal.

The media have reported numerous cases of suspected hGH use as a performance enhancer. For example, Inge de Bruijn, a Dutch swimmer who set four world records, was accused of taking hGH (*Boston Globe*, September 22, 2000); an Usbeki coach was caught with a stash of hGH (*Christian Science Monitor*, September 12, 2000); a Chinese swimmer on her way to a competition was detained at Perth airport with thirteen vials of hGH in her thermos (Zorpette, 2000); and a potential baseball scandal connected hGH and steroid use to some of the game's biggest stars (Fainaru-Wada and Williams, 2006). None of these cases yet compares with the widespread use of steroids by the East Europeans or the media coverage given to Ben Johnson's being stripped of his gold medal for the 100-meter run after failing a drug test, but the reports are surely only the tip of the iceberg. Tests for hGH were administered for the first time during the 2004 Athens Olympics, although there are questions as to whether the tests can adequately detect the substance (Sallah, 2004).

THE FACES OF BIOMEDICAL ENHANCEMENT

Some forms of intervention are administered in order to treat generally accepted medical diseases. Treating human growth hormone deficiency with hGH is an example of such intervention. Short children who cannot produce enough hGH on their own are treated with the hormone, just as people with diabetes are treated with insulin. But the line between therapy and enhancement is thin.

As we know from earlier studies of medicalization (Conrad, 1992, 2000), a wide range of conditions or behaviors can be defined as a medical problem, as some kind of disorder in need of treatment. We also know that conditions can move in and out of medical jurisdiction. Medical definitions can change; new medical diagnoses can be developed that will justify certain types of enhancement as therapy. As noted in chapter 3, adult ADHD has become a common diagnosis, and Ritalin is often prescribed for it. In a recent article the chief of Mental Health Services at Harvard noted that stimulants are widely used among college students to "get an edge" (Kadison, 2005). Many "successful" adults, citing problems with personal disorganization or an inability to finish projects, have diagnosed themselves as having ADHD and sought treatment from physicians. Much of this Ritalin use may actually be an enhancement rather than a treatment; hence I have called it a "medicalization of underperformance." Rudman's definition of "growth hormone menopause," deemed to cause the bodily deterioration of aging (Foreman, 1992), might be considered another example of expanding therapeutic justification. While there are certainly disorders for which there is general agreement that a biological disease exists, there are also many disorders that are contestable or controversial.

In the discussion thus far we have seen that hCH is used as a biomedical solution to what are fundamentally social problems: shortness, aging, and athletic edge. But these examples also provide us with the opportunity to examine the different faces of biomedical enhancement. As noted earlier, in my view, enhancement is an intervention that takes the body or performance to where it has never been before. In this section I conceptualize three different, though related, faces of enhancement: normalization, repair, and performance edge.

Normalization

When biomedical enhancements are used with the goal of bringing the body into line with what the physician or patient deems to be the "normal" or socially expected standard, this type of enhancement can be called "normalization"; an alternative term might be "standardization." Normalization occurs, for example, when parents of idiopathically short children approach the medical system requesting hGH treatments or when doctors suggest medical treatments for shortness. The goal is to reach or get closer to the normal (i.e., average) height of the population.

There are other examples of normalizing biomedical enhancement. At different times, women have sought to enlarge or reduce the size of their breasts, based on the prevailing social convention (Yalom, 1997). In recent years some women have sought surgical breast augmentation to bring their bodies into line with some kind of social ideal of feminine beauty (Haiken, 1997; Jacobson, 2000). One study of women who underwent plastic surgery suggests that the intervention allows women to "successfully reposition their bodies as 'normal' bodies, giving them the body they were meant to have" (Gimlin, 2000: 77). When physicians define small breasts as "micromastia," as some did in the 1950s, they facilitate the medicalization of enhancement (Jacobson, 2000: 66).

Other examples of normalization include plastic surgery to make Asian women's eyes more oval or "Western" in shape (Kaw, 1992) and rhinoplasty to reshape "ethnic-looking" noses. All these efforts are attempts to enhance the body to meet some kind of cultural standard or ideal. In American society, the perceived standard of Anglo-Saxon beauty and youthful appearance dictates the types of enhancement that are currently desirable.

Repair

Many forms of enhancement involve the use of biomedical interventions to rejuvenate the body or restore it to a previous condition. The use of hGH to relieve some of the effects of aging is a good example. The goal of such intervention (regardless of its actual efficacy) is to repair the body, to restore muscle, improve skin, and lose fat. Many forms of cosmetic surgery also represent this type of enhancement. Facelifts, tummy tucks, and liposuction often represent an attempt to regain youth. In this context, Viagra can be deemed an enhancement as well, especially as it attempts to restore sexual performance to a previous level. In each of these cases a biomedical enhancement is used to repair some bodily malfunction or misshapen body part.

Such enhancements can also be regarded as an attempt "to repair the disjunction that can develop between the internal and the external" (Haiken, 2000: 88). Many who have undergone cosmetic surgery say that the surgery has aligned their body with their identity. Transsexual or transgender operations exemplify a somewhat different type of "repair," whereby the surgery is done to align the body with the individual's identity (cf. H. Rubin, 2003). In this case the intervention does not return the body to a previous condition but rather takes it to a place it has never been before.

Performance Edge

Most biomedical enhancements attempt to alter the body, but others focus directly on performance. In recent years biomedical interventions have been added to the armamentarium of rigorous training, special diets, potions, and life regimens as methods to improve athletic performance. Steroids have been the most widely used of the performance-enhancing drugs, but in the past decade hGH has also become a drug of choice. In organized professional and amateur sports, such drugs have been made illegal, and doping has become a major social problem in the Olympics and elsewhere. But there is no doubt that the pressures of competition can lead some athletes to seek biomedical enhancements to improve their performance.

Athletes are not the only ones who use prescription drugs for enhancement. Some people use Prozac and similar medications to aid them in their pursuit of happiness (Elliott, 1999). Other drugs such as Ritalin for adult ADHD, beta blockers for "stage fright" (D. Harris, 2001), or Paxil for shyness (Meyer, 1996; S. Scott, 2006) may also be seen as performance enhancers. A widening array of people see prescription drugs as a legitimate way to improve life performance.

In most cases of enhancement, context is important. Expanding on an example mentioned earlier, taking a cognitive drug for the treatment of Alzheimer disease is a therapy, while taking it for "senior moments" is something of a repair; taking it to improve an SAT score might be considered an acceptable enhancement, while taking it prior to a chess match might be deemed a form of doping that makes the competition unfair (see Frankford, 1998: 71). So the enhancement inheres not in the biomedical composition of the intervention but in when and how it is used.

THE TEMPTATIONS OF BIOMEDICAL ENHANCEMENT

The quest for a more voluptuous body, the fascination with eternal youth, and the pursuit of athletic victory are long-held and deeply ingrained social and individual goals in American culture. Such goals are not unusual in a culture that values bigger, faster, and more; they are but three desires among many such. The contours of these desires may vary with fashion—small breasts and large breasts were each idealized in different eras—but the cultural goal of reshaping the body endures (cf. Conrad and Jacobson, 2003).

Attaining these objectives is socially rewarded, and there are many routes toward achieving them. The process typically involves hard work and dedication to a task but may also entail specific techniques, special potions, or even magical incantations. Along the way, charlatans may promise special keys to achieving these goals but leave the seeker disappointed and feeling cheated.

In this context, the temptations of biomedical enhancements provide an inducement for individuals and groups to modify their situation. Sociologists seldom use the term "temptation" when referring to motivation or social phenomena (cf. Toby, 1998), perhaps because of its moral connotation as an enticement toward evil or sin (see *Oxford English Dictionary*). However, I use the term here in a morally neutral way to mean something that is attractive, alluring, or inviting toward some action or goal, regardless of its moral evaluation. In a sense, biomedical enhancement is a double temptation: the object itself (e.g., several inches of height, younger features, improved performance) is tempting, and so is the biomedical route toward that object (e.g., a rapid means to improvement, a new technological strategy, a medical solution).

Enhancements are a social temptation in that they can create a competitive difference among otherwise similar individuals. They offer a personal advantage, and society will reward those who have an edge (D. Rothman, 2001). The key to the notion of enhancement, however, is that only some are enhanced. There is no edge if the attribute is universal. Consider a biomedical enhancement that would add 6 inches to height. If it were available to only a limited number of individuals, it would certainly increase their height and perhaps enhance their life opportunities (for social acceptance and perhaps especially for basketball). But if this enhancement were widely available and most people availed themselves of it, it would no longer provide a competitive advantage. The situation would be like that of the mythical town of Lake Wobegon, where all the children are above average. In reality, although a short person would be 6 inches taller, virtually everyone else would also be 6 inches taller, and the shorter person would still be short. Maintaining the edge of enhancement requires that only a few may be enhanced.

If most people are enhanced, then the intervention is no longer an enhancement but becomes a necessity. One interesting nonmedical example would be "test preparation" courses (marketed in the United States under the name Stanley Kaplan or Princeton Review) for the American medical school admissions test (MCAT). Forty years ago, only a small percentage of students took test preparation courses to prepare for the MCAT; it was an enhancement and provided a competitive edge. Today, such a high percentage of students take prep courses that not to take the course puts students at a disadvantage. Thus, when everyone, or even a large proportion of a population, is enhanced, the advantages of enhancement are severely altered and temptation gives way to requirement. A highly successful enhancement can create a market for itself and become a virtual necessity.

The social forces driving biomedical enhancement are strong. As David Rothman (2001) points out, there are powerful engines of enhancement, including science, medicine, commerce, and culture. Science and medicine work to create new treatments for human problems, some of which may become enhancements. As Eric Juengst notes, "All interventions that will come to be used as treatments for sick people will also be posed as enhancements for well people" (1998: 43). Prozac was first introduced for the clinically depressed but was soon touted as a means to make individuals better than well (Elliott, 2003); it is likely that treatments for Alzheimer disease will lead to memory enhancements for the rest of us (Hall, 2003). As with hGH, these interventions are first legitimized for medical problems, then later are promoted to enhance nonmedical conditions. The biotechnology industry is fueled by a partnership between science and commerce; it produces new interventions (e.g., pharmaceutical, genetic) and finds or creates markets for them. As noted earlier, in numerous areas there already exists a cultural demand for a potential enhancement (e.g., hGH or breast augmentation), so the market is already there. Forms of repair and normalization may be in the front line and may lead to increased enhancements; in 1998, 2 million Americans elected to undergo medical cosmetic procedures (Haiken, 2000: 83). According to the website of the American Society for Aesthetic Plastic Surgery, 11.5 million cosmetic surgical *procedures* were performed in 2005 (ASAPS, 2005b). Given the aging of our population and the antiaging sentiments prevalent in our culture, it is not surprising to see an expanding biomedical repair market. While there are constraints to the implementation of biomedical enhancements, including questions of efficacy, the "risks" of use (Rothman, 2001), the cost, and the potential for government regulation (Mehlman, 2000), our society presents a fertile ground for the development of biomedical enhancements.

THE DILEMMAS OF BIOMEDICAL ENHANCEMENT

Efficacy is one of the most obvious issues of biomedical enhancement. Does the intervention accomplish what it is intended to do? Do consumers get improvement for their investment, or are they being fooled? While this is a significant issue, it does not directly concern us here. Many enhancements continue to be sought despite a lack of evidence for their success. Consider the various potions and nostrums that have been promoted throughout history for increasing sexual potency; the fact that most (if not all) performed no better than placebos neither dampened the search nor discouraged the use of a whole range of elixirs (H. Green, 1986). I will bracket the issue of efficacy here and discuss some social issues that are inherent in biomedical enhancement regardless of efficacy.

Is Biomedical Enhancement Unnatural?

Questions are often raised as to whether biomedical enhancements are "unnatural." Does modifying height by taking hGH or augmenting breast size with cosmetic surgery constitute using medical interventions to enhance what would otherwise be one's "natural," smaller, characteristics? Taking medicine or having surgery to modify one's features imparts, some would say, a "taint of inauthenticity" to these improvements (Gimlin, 2000).

The term "natural" is often taken as a proxy for "good." Natural foods are better than processed foods, natural fibers better than chemical fibers, and so on. But smallpox is natural and the vaccine to prevent it is not; poisonous mushrooms and annoying allergies are also natural. There is no necessary moral value to being natural, nor is the unnatural intrinsically inauthentic or second-rate.

Perhaps the negative evaluation of unnatural enhancements comes from another, more social, source. The power of the Protestant ethic has long been recognized in our society. As Max Weber (1904/1958) observed, in our Calvinist-based culture we must work hard in order to show that we are among those who will attain salvation. Biomedical enhancements do not involve hard work; in fact they are something of a technological fix. Most people probably do not deem "unnatural" the muscle tone of fitness buffs who work out ten hours a week or the aerobic ability of marathon runners. Indeed, we admire such individuals for their fortitude. They have achieved their enhancement through diligence and hard work, exemplary characteristics in our culture. If women could enhance their breasts at the gym or children increase their height by working out, would naturalness be an issue at all? Our society has adopted a sort of "pharmacological Calvinism" when it comes to taking medications (Klerman, 1972). That is, we believe it is better to achieve an objective such as pleasure, sexual satisfaction, mental stability, and bodily fitness naturally than with drugs or medications. Using drugs is an inferior and even suspect way of reaching a goal. But what is natural resides in the social definition, not in the phenomenon.

A Question of Fairness?

Biomedical enhancements can provide an advantage or a competitive edge for an individual. This is most apparent in athletics, but it is also inherent in most forms of enhancement. In athletic competition, performance enhancements are seen as giving someone an unfair edge; use is deemed a form of cheating and is severely sanctioned by various athletic authorities. Drug enhancements are a huge problem in the Olympics, and a significant problem for most professional sports. But what constitutes an illegitimate enhancement is subject to definition. In the United States, when baseball star Mark McGuire hit seventy home runs, breaking Roger Maris's record, it was widely reported that he took Andro (androstenedoine). Though proven to increase testosterone, Andro was considered a supplement. Had McGuire been playing in the National Football League, on a college athletic team, or participating in the Olympics, he would have been sanctioned for taking a prohibited steroid substance. What in one setting is merely a supplement becomes in another an illegal enhancement. (McGuire was later accused of taking steroids in addition to Andro, but the point here is the variability about what is labeled an illegal enhancement.)

Fairness is also at issue when only a limited number of people or competitors have access to an enhancement. If all runners took steroids, would fairness be at issue? To take another example from sports, forty years ago bamboo or metal poles were standard fare for pole vaulting; in the late 1960s, fiberglass poles (which had greater elasticity) were introduced, giving an enormous advantage to those who used them. Suddenly vaulters were soaring to new heights. But the fiberglass pole was not prohibited as an enhancement; rather, it was embraced as the new way to compete in the sport. If some drug had put the extra spring in the vaulters' legs to set these same records, would the use of this drug have been defined as unfair and illegitimate, even if it could have been made available to all competitors?

One of the most fundamental fairness issues is that most biomedical enhancements are not available to everybody. These limitations make their use frequently élitist. Usually their use will reflect the distribution of resources in society; those with the greatest resources are most likely to be able to afford the cost or have access to biomedicine. The cost of hGH is likely to limit its availability to those who have $20,000 per year to invest in the height of their children or to those who can purchase it to improve their athletic performance. By and large, health insurance in the United States does not cover most enhancements, although it reimburses some of what we call therapy or repair (such as memory drugs for Alzheimer disease or Viagra for sexual dysfunction). Some contend that this coverage is a slippery slope toward supporting consumers' desires for enhancements for the sake of normalization or improved performance. And even if biomedical enhancements were covered by insurance, a question of fairness still remains for 44 million Americans without health insurance.

The invisibility of biomedical enhancements is perhaps one of their greatest threats to fairness. This is certainly the case in sports competition; it may be manifested as inauthenticity with other enhanced characteristics. After all, someone could be enhanced with none of the other competitors knowing it. This lack of knowledge gives the enhanced competitor an unknown and undetected advantage. If the benefit were known, could one take this advantage into account? Would this reduce the unfairness? Thus, drug testing becomes important in the attempt to maintain a level playing field, although other advantages that may depend on unequal resources (like training facilities, economic support, or coaching) are not deemed unfair enhancements.[5] It is also interesting that we seldom hear complaints about symphony orchestra players having an unfair advantage if they take beta blockers for stage fright before a big concert.

Issues of Risk and Permanence

As David Rothman (2001) notes, what is an acceptable risk for treatment of disease may not be an acceptable risk for enhancement. Risks can either be medical or social. The composer Robert Schumann used a mechanical device to extend his fingers so as to become a better pianist, causing a permanent numbness in the middle finger of his right hand (Sadie and Tyrrell, 2001: 761). We have numerous examples of medical risks: increased cancer risk or possibility of rupture with silicone breast implants; higher rates of pancreatic cancer and heart disease as well as shutdown of testosterone production with steroid use; risk of high blood pressure, diabetes, or heart disease with hGH (Fackelmann, 1990). Unpleasant side effects can also accompany these enhancements: calcium deposits and hardening of scar tissue that causes pain and disfigurement from silicone breast implants; unwanted breast enlargement (in both men and women) and stunted growth in adolescents from steroid use; sexual dysfunction from Prozac; and heightened cholesterol, increased blood pressure, joint pain, carpel tunnel syndrome, or swollen ankles from hGH (Papadakis et al., 1996; C. Johnson, 2006).

There are social risks as well. As noted earlier, enhancements can reinforce the social values that prompted them in the first place. For example, the use of hGH reaffirms perceptions about the importance of height or the undesirable attributes of aging bodies. Enhancements allow an individual to try to become someone he or she is not (e.g., to try to pass as a younger person) and so may create risks to identity as well. Finally, enhancements may entail the risk of discovery. The athlete who uses hGH or steroids, the breast-augmented woman who wants to be seen as natural, the man who has had a hair implant and a face lift in order to pass himself off as youthful—they all live in fear of disclosure. The veneer of authenticity is always a risk.

One of the unique features of many biomedical enhancements when compared with other enhancements is their apparent permanency (enhancements achieved through drugs are an exception). The perception is that once a biomedical enhancement has been implemented, it cannot be altered. One cannot undo the inches gained from hGH treatment or return a nose to its original shape, though breast implants can be removed and the results of many types of cosmetic surgery can be altered again. (It should be noted, however, that this apparent reversal does not necessarily return the body to its prior condition; frequently some damage has occurred in the process.) One can even ask whether social enhancements like learning the violin or mastering a foreign language are any less permanent than a few inches of height. While it is true that biomedical enhancements may be more difficult to reverse than social enhancements (and this would be true for such minor modifications as tattoos as well), most are not of the permanent variety (although the inherent risks and sequelae might persist). It is likely that if genetic enhancements were available, permanence might be much more of an issue.

Shifting Social Meanings

The message that biomedical enhancements impart is that individuals are dissatisfied with their current condition, whether it be height, breast size, or performance. Dealing with this dissatisfaction through biomedical means, however, may be seen as a profoundly individual approach. Rather than attempting to change the definition of the condition or problem at hand, the biomedical approach endeavors to enhance the individual up to or beyond a targeted standard. In this sense biomedical enhancements are inherently conservative strategies: they change the individual rather than deal with the social standard or expectation in a more collective manner.

Using biomedical enhancements may perpetuate a sense of inadequacy. When one opts for using hGH to increase height, for example, one is complicit with whatever heightism exists in society; the biomedical enhancement validates the belief that shortness is undesirable and should be changed. It reinforces the stigma of shortness, and at the same time it potentially reduces societal diversity. When a socially constructed standard, like 6-foot-tall men or size 36C breasts, comes to be seen as an important vehicle for success, the temptations to attain this standard may increase. If a significant number of people use enhancements to achieve a certain goal, then the enhancement has the potential to decrease the diversity in society. People will make their bodies more similar, with the same height or breast size. For the moment, the impact of biomedical enhancements is a statistical blip, but the potential remains. How, then, will this affect the social standard?

IS BETTER ALWAYS GOOD?

Human growth hormone provides us with a window through which to examine biomedical enhancement. We have seen that hGH has been touted as a potential enhancement for idiopathic shortness, as an antiaging agent, and as an athletic performance enhancement. Bracketing the question of efficacy, claims for hGH's enhancement potential have been widely circulated in various social realms.[6]

The interest in hGH as a biomedical enhancement stems from the production in 1985 of synthetic hGH, which made it cheaper and more easily available. At first the drug companies advertised hGH for FDA-approved uses, primarily for children with human growth hormone deficiency. Following this development, physicians, patients, and drug companies all sought other medical uses for hGH. Some physicians began promoting it for other "problems," medicalizing idiopathic short stature and aging bodies. If hGH could be used to increase the height of all children in the lowest three percentiles, the potential markets would expand enormously. Off-label uses of hGH were so common that Congress investigated whether drug companies were promoting hGH for applications that were not FDA approved. In recent years, off-label restrictions have been eased, allowing drug manufacturers to disseminate information on off-label uses, so long as balanced and scientific evidence is presented. The actual scientific evidence for height enhancement of children without hormone deficiency is equivocal, with some small gains possible; the evidence that it functions as an antiaging agent has been refuted, and there has been no research on hGH and performance enhancement. Off-label claims for hGH continue in doctors' offices, on the Internet, and in various subcultures. The demand for the kinds of improvement that the drug can bring has not faltered, and the hopes for biomedical enhancement remain. Sales of hGH in 2004 totaled $622 million (C. Johnson, 2006).

Considering hGH as a case of biomedical enhancement allows us to raise some broader issues. In the first place, we can now see that biomedical enhancements have several faces, including normalization, augmentation, and repair. These categories may be useful for understanding the uses of enhancements in different situations. Here, however, I want briefly to look at a few issues that may apply in any biomedical enhancement. There are numerous ways of subdividing what we are calling biomedical enhancements. Some, for example, may require medicalization of the problem prior to intervention. This is true for enhancements delivered by the medical profession (e.g., cosmetic surgery, treatments with medication). But some biomedical enhancements occur outside professional medical jurisdiction, although they are still considered "medical" types of intervention. These include biomedical supplements like hGH that can be purchased over the Internet or on the black market for enhancing athletic performance.

The legitimacy of a biomedical enhancement depends in part on the viewpoint one adopts. Chapters in recent books point to some contentious policy issues: Allen Buchanan and his colleagues (2000) ask, "Why not the best?" while Erik Parens (1998) counters with, "Is better always good?" We can bracket the specific ethical issues these authors raise and yet appreciate that these questions capture fundamental questions raised by biomedical enhancements. In our achievement-oriented society one can justifiably ask, Why *not* seek the best in all ways possible within ethical and legal limits? But the cultural assumption that better is always good needs to be questioned. Simply because there is a demand for enhancement and the technology to do it does not mean that the result is always beneficial, particularly for society. Issues such as risk, fairness, equity, authenticity, and individual choice loom large. A reservoir of cultural ambivalence about biomedical enhancements is reflected in popular films like *Gattaca* (1997) and skeptical treatises like the recent *Better Than Well* (Elliott, 2003). As philosophers have argued for centuries, individual benefit may conflict with the public good. The potential of genetic enhancement extends and amplifies these issues.

Biomedical enhancement may be most developed in twenty-first-century America, but aspects of it are certainly evident elsewhere. It resides at the crossroads of our cultural belief in self-improvement, an individual's desire to get ahead of the competition, our faith in medical solutions to human problems, and the economic drive and market-making of the biotechnology industry. The wellspring of biomedical enhancement is embedded in the very fabric of our society, and science and medicine will provide us with even greater technologies for "improvement" in the future. We must recognize the social and cultural impacts of biomedical enhancements so that we can better deal with the temptations that are sure to come.

CHAPTER FIVE

Continuity

Homosexuality and the Potential for Remedicalization

Demedicalization occurs when a problem is no longer defined in medical terms and the involvement of medical personnel is no longer deemed appropriate. There are only a few documented examples of almost complete demedicalization; these include masturbation (Engelhardt, 1974) and homosexuality (Conrad and Schneider, 1992). Masturbation was first defined as a sin (the sin of Onan), then as a moral weakness. During the Victorian era it became defined as an illness; there is a huge literature on masturbatory insanity and on the disease of "self-abuse." Under Freud's influence only compulsive masturbation was deemed a clinical problem. When Kinsey found that more than 90 percent of men masturbated, the practice became at least statistically normal, and with the work of sexologists Masters and Johnson in the 1960s, masturbation came to be regarded as healthy and those who didn't masturbate were seen as sexually repressed. Whatever the behavior is, masturbation probably didn't change, but the definition and social response to it did change (Engelhardt, 1974).

Like masturbation, homosexuality is an example of almost complete demedicalization. This chapter examines changes that may have affected or modified the demedicalization of homosexuality in the last thirty years. After briefly reviewing the medicalization and demedicalization of homosexuality, I explore four areas where changes may have affected demedicalization: (1) shifts and developments in psychiatry; (2) the emergence of HIV/AIDS; (3) discoveries in genetics; and (4) changes in conception and language in the gay community. I conclude with a reassessment of demedicalization and the potential for the remedicalization of homosexual conduct.

EMERGING MEDICAL CONCEPTIONS
OF MALE HOMOSEXUALITY: A REVIEW

The roots of the medicalization of male homosexuality can be found in the mid-nineteenth century, in the context of severe criminalization of homosexual conduct. The term "homosexuality" was coined in 1869 by Hungarian physician K. M. Benkert, who argued against the repressive laws and harsh punishments of the Prussian legal code. He contended that such treatment was unjust and ineffective because homosexuality was congenital rather than acquired (Conrad and Schneider, 1992). He defined homosexuality as a medical pathology rather than a criminal offense. Perhaps the most important nineteenth-century medical figure in this regard was Richard Kraft-Ebbing, a German physician-psychiatrist who wrote *Psychopathia Sexualis*, a monumental work on "sexual abnormalities" published in 1886. Kraft-Ebbing suggested that most cases of "sexual inversion" (his term for homosexuality) result from a congenital weakness in the nervous system. He argued that homosexuals could not change the direction or the expression of their sexual desires and therefore should be treated therapeutically rather than punitively. He called not for sympathy, but understanding (Conrad and Schneider, 1992: 184). Thus, the original medicalization of homosexuality was meant as a form of protection against oppressive legal sanctions, although oppressive medical practices still emerged in psychiatric attempts to change homosexuals into heterosexuals.

In the early twentieth century, Sigmund Freud revolutionized the way medicine and psychiatry defined and treated a wide range of human problems. He explained homosexuality in terms of his general theory of sexuality and rejected notions of a congenital etiology. He saw homoerotic desires as a part of normal child development that must be abandoned or "repressed" for the sake of "mature" adult development. Although homosexuality was an undesirable state, in his view, it was linked to "normal" sexual development and was a "variation" rather than a disease or disorder. Freud was not optimistic that homosexuality could be changed by medical treatment or psychoanalysis. (For a detailed discussion, see Conrad and Schneider, 1992: 185–87; Terry, 1999.)

Freud's followers, however, took a different tack. They reestablished homosexuality as a psychiatric pathology and claimed to possess a treatment that could be a cure. Beginning in the 1940s, three practicing psychiatrists, all adopting some variation of Freudian psychodynamic theory, emerged as the most influential American advocates of the homosexuality-as-illness perspective: Edmund Bergler, Irving Bieber, and Charles Socarides. Bergler's 1956 book *Homosexuality: Disease or Way of Life?* presented a distinctly negative portrait (e.g., describing homosexuals as "megaloma-

niacal" individuals exhibiting "free floating malice," "unreliability," and "supercil-
iousness") and insisted that all homosexuals experienced a deep sense of guilt over
their "perversion," which was at its root a disease. Bieber and his colleagues presented a more ambitious psychoanalytic defense of homosexuality as a pathology in
their 1962 book, *Homosexuality: A Psychoanalytic Study*. It was based on a comparative study of 100 homosexuals and heterosexuals under psychiatric treatment.
While more reserved in its moral tone than Bergler's book, Bieber's work characterized homosexuality as a pathology rooted in flawed childhood and family relationships. Socarides has been an active and vocal advocate of the pathological perspective on homosexuality. From his 1968 book *The Overt Homosexual* to his current
websites, he remains one of the staunchest defenders of the notion of homosexuality as a serious medical pathology. For him, like Bergler and Bieber, homosexuality
is a form of mental illness with "pre-Oedipal" origins. All believed in the efficacy of
psychoanalytic treatment for changing homosexuals into heterosexuals—at least in
some cases. (For more on this subject, see Conrad and Schneider, 1992: 172–213.)

The final piece necessary for the medicalization of homosexuality was its inclusion in the American Psychiatric Association's official classification of psychiatric
disorders, the *Diagnostic and Statistical Manual of Mental Disorders*, and its parent
document, the World Health Organization's *International Classification of Diseases*
(WHO, 1994). These volumes represent the professionally approved definitions and
diagnostic labels for virtually all mental disorders that concern psychiatry. For our
purposes here, I focus on the DSM. While homosexuality was mentioned in the
1952 edition, known as DSM-I (APA, 1952), the DSM-II (APA, 1968) clearly defined
it as a medical pathology. Without offering a specific definition of what constitutes
the "condition," the DSM-II categorized homosexuality under "Personality Disorders and *Certain* Other Non-Psychotic Disorders," specifically under "Sexual Devi-
ation." Homosexuality was now an official mental disorder, a psychopathology. But
this definition would soon be challenged.

There is a long history of advocates and researchers who claim that homosexuality,
while perhaps congenital, is not pathological. (For a detailed review of the context of
the demedicalization of homosexuality, see Conrad and Schneider, 1992: 193–209.) Although the seeds of protest were planted earlier, the most immediate agent in this
changing view was the "gay liberation" movement of the late 1960s. Shaped by the 1969
Stonewall protests in Greenwich Village, a gay social movement emerged that demanded an end to persecution and discrimination, fought to establish gay civil rights,
and adopted militant and confrontational tactics when necessary. Led by two organizations, the Gay Liberation Front and the Gay Activist Alliance, the movement sought
to locate sources of oppression of gays and to develop strategies to combat them.

The new self-definition of "gay pride," which essentially presented the image of the "healthy homosexual," contradicted both the official medical view and the public statements of a handful of vocal psychiatric opponents (Conrad and Schneider, 1992: 203). With a combination of direct actions and disruptions at professional conferences (called "zapping"), public challenges to the main proponents of the medical view (especially Bieber and Socarides), and negotiation in the committees that were revising the DSM, gay activists and their allies set out to change the psychiatric definition and treatment of homosexuality.

The activists had some support within the profession for removing homosexuality from the DSM. By carefully evaluating and criticizing the scientific evidence for the disease model, they convinced the APA nomenclature committee that some change in classification was needed. The committee compromised, revising the DSM so that homosexuality by itself was not a diagnosis or illness; only those individuals who were unhappy with their sexual orientation were said to have a disorder. The resolution was accepted by the APA Board of Trustees in December 1973, and a few months later it passed by APA vote. The new diagnosis, "sexual orientation disturbance (homosexuality)," would replace the existing medicalized definition of homosexuality. Homosexuality had been demedicalized and, at least officially, was no longer to be considered an illness (cf. Stevens and Hall, 1991; Bayer, 1987; Conrad and Schneider, 1992: 172–213).

Although it is unclear how much the demedicalization itself improved the lives of gay men and women, it was clearly a symbolic victory. A major professional association had voted the disease of homosexuality out of existence; homosexuals were no longer officially deemed sick, and this was public knowledge.

DEMEDICALIZATION AND FOUR ARENAS OF CHANGE

Since 1974, numerous changes may have affected the demedicalization of homosexuality. In this section I examine aspects of four arenas of change as they relate to the medical definitions and treatment of homosexual conduct: (1) psychiatry; (2) treatment of HIV/AIDS; (3) genetics; and (4) changing perceptions in the gay community.

Transformations in Psychiatry

Since the 1973 APA decision, several changes within psychiatry have affected medical conceptions of homosexuality. First, biomedical psychiatry became dominant, overtaking psychoanalytic approaches. Increasingly, decisions about revisions to the DSM were based on purported scientific evidence rather than on theoretical agendas (Kirk and Kutchins, 1992: 7; Horwitz, 2002). Second, the gay rights movement and subsequent gay, lesbian, bisexual, and transgender (GLBT) organizations stimulated the development of gay and lesbian advocacy groups within psychiatry, psychology, and social work, including the APA (Krajeski, 1996: 28). Both of these forces encouraged the continued demedicalization of adult homosexuality. Many activists, however, have claimed that the emergence of "gender identity disorder" may create a backdoor to remedicalization.

The Rise and Fall of "Ego-Dystonic Homosexuality"

Despite the 1974 decision, the diagnosis "sexual orientation disturbance" remained in the DSM for the purpose of treating gays and lesbians who were conflicted about their sexuality and/or interested in developing a heterosexual orientation (Campbell, 1983: 29). While gay and lesbian activists both within psychiatry and outside it were opposed to the residual diagnosis, they felt protest would draw attention to the fact that homosexuality had not been completely removed from the psychiatric manual and thus dilute the political victory (Kutchins and Kirk, 1997: 78). In the context of the development of the DSM-III, however, a debate around the residual diagnosis occurred. The diagnosis morphed through several names (Bayer, 1987; Sultan, Elsner, and Smith, 1987) before emerging as "ego-dystonic homosexuality" (EDH) in the DSM-III (1980). This "compromise" diagnosis (Kutchins and Kirk, 1997: 90) changed the emphasis from conflict about sexual orientation to the inability to achieve heterosexual arousal. The EDH diagnosis in the DSM-III states, "This category is reserved for those homosexuals for whom changing sexual orientations is a persistent concern, and should be avoided in cases where the desire to change sexual orientations may be a brief, temporary manifestation of an individual's difficulty in adjusting to a new awareness of his or her homosexual impulses" (APA, 1980: 281). Some gay activists in psychiatry opposed the inclusion of EDH because they believed that it continued to present heterosexuality as preferable, while others believed that it retained homosexuality in the DSM, albeit in a modified form (Bayer, 1987; Kutchins and Kirk, 1997).

The EDH diagnosis was short-lived. During the 1980s the diagnosis was seldom used, and research on the disorder was limited (Diamont, 1987). Gay activists and supporters within psychiatry (e.g., the Association of Gay and Lesbian Psychiatrists) felt that the diagnosis continued to pathologize homosexuality and lobbied for its removal from the next revision of the DSM. Again, after significant investigation and debate, the committees representing gay activist viewpoints won the day (Bayer, 1987; Kutchins and Kirk, 1997) and EDH was dropped from the DSM-III-R (1987).

One of the last vestiges of medicalized homosexuality was removed from psychiatry's official manual. (See Kutchins and Kirk, 1997.)

The Emergence of NARTH and GID

At least two other factors may affect the demedicalization of homosexuality: the development of an organization that promotes the medical treatment of homosexuality and the emergence of a diagnosis that describes deviations in children's gender identity.

Despite the demise of EDH, a small but vocal group of psychiatrists continues to offer reparative or conversion therapy for gays and lesbians (Cohler and Galatzer-Levy, 2000: 340–52). The most vocal claims-makers for the pathological view of homosexuality are a group of psychoanalysts called the National Association for Research and Therapy of Homosexuality. NARTH, established in 1992, is led by Charles Socarides and Joseph Nicolosi. Socarides was an advocate for the retention of the homosexuality diagnosis in the DSM-II in the 1970s. Central to both Nicolosi's and Socarides's claims is a belief that homosexuality is a result of an unhealthy childhood development, thus not biological and therefore changeable. NARTH formed strategic alliances with conservative family and religious organizations, promoting the notion that homosexuality is "curable" with conversion therapy. They defend conversion therapy with civil rights rhetoric, contending that gays and lesbians who are distressed about their sexuality should have the "liberty" to choose treatment (Kutchins and Kirk, 1997: 93–94). Members of NARTH have not developed sufficient professional or political power to influence the psychiatric definition of homosexuality, but they continue to champion for the remedicalization of homosexuality in and out of psychiatry (see www.narth.com).

The diagnosis of "gender identity disorder" (GID) was placed in the DSM-III in 1980 to allow for the treatment of (1) transgender and transsexual adults and (2) children who exhibit pervasive cross-gender behavior and discomfort about their sex organs. Twenty years of research on conflicting and ambiguous sex and gender roles by researchers Richard Green and John Money led to its inclusion (Green and Money, 1960; Zucker, 1990). The current debate relating to the etiology of homosexuality turns on the diagnosis of children and research claims that the majority of children treated for GID grow up to be gay or bisexual adults. Opponents of the diagnosis claim that the disorder is medicalizing the normal development of gays and lesbians.

The description of the diagnosis in the DSM-IV-TR (2000) represents the APA's current statement on the disorder. The diagnosis under the heading "sexual and gender identity disorders" (APA, 2000: 535) emphasizes the role of gender and can

be applied to children, adults, or adolescents. According to the DSM-IV-TR, to diagnose a child with GID:

> There must be evidence of a strong and persistent cross-gender identification, which is
> the desire to be, or the insistence that one is, of the other sex (Criterion A). This cross-
> gender identification must not merely be a desire for any perceived cultural advantages
> of being the other sex. There must also be evidence of persistent discomfort about one's
> assigned sex or a sense of inappropriateness in the gender role of that sex (Criterion
> B). . . . To make the diagnosis, there must be evidence of clinically significant distress
> or impairment in social, occupational, or other important areas of functioning (Crite-
> rion D). [APA, 2000: 576]

The rallying point for the debates over GID concerns scientific evidence suggesting that a majority of children, particularly boys, who are diagnosed with GID
become gay or bisexual. A pinnacle study was Richard Green's *The "Sissy Boy Syndrome" and the Development of Homosexuality* (1987). Green followed a group of
44 boys diagnosed with GID until adolescence. He found that 33 (75%) of the boys
developed bisexual or homosexual desires. Other scholars have found some evidence correlating GID with adult homosexuality (see Zucker, 1990). Some psychiatrists see GID as a normal stage for homosexual development and argue that it
should be deleted from the DSM (Isay, 2002). In the context of contested evidence,
even if a significant proportion of boys with GID grow up to be gay, most gays and
lesbians are never diagnosed with GID.

Among the supporters of the GID diagnosis are the APA, some health practitioners prominent in the field of sexual and gender disorders (e.g., Zucker and
Bradley, 1995), NARTH, and some transsexuals who are concerned about reim-
bursement for sex-reassignment surgery. Most interesting here are members of the
transsexual community who argue that insurance companies would refuse to pay for
sex-change operations if the diagnosis were dropped.

While not all the proponents of the GID diagnosis emphasize the relationship
between childhood GID and adult homosexuality, the critics are concerned with
the alleged "prehomosexual behavior" as a pathology (Zucker and Bradley, 1995).
Even the most ardent critics of the diagnosis, however, lobby for gender identity "reform" rather than removal; they propose the demedicalization of GID in childhood
but allow for some form of medicalized transsexualism to enable sex-change operations (e.g., www.GIDreform.org). Psychiatrist Richard Isay is the foremost propo-
nent that GID is not a pathology but a normal stage in homosexual development.
He sees GID as a "vestige" of the medicalization of homosexuality and believes that
the diagnosis "implicitly labels homosexual boys as mentally disordered" (2002: 1).

Signaling the strength of the GID reform movement within the APA, the Committee on Gay, Lesbian, and Bisexual Issues demanded a reevaluation of the childhood GID diagnosis in 1997. In support, the Gay and Lesbian Medical Association advocated the creation of a task force within the APA to investigate childhood GID and develop revisions for the 2000 edition of the DSM (Isay, 2002). Despite such calls to action, the GID diagnosis was not significantly revised for the DSM-IV-TR (2000). That GLBT organizations both outside and inside the medical community advocate GID reform, however, signifies the growing strength of the GID reform movement and may allow for the demedicalization of the diagnosis in future years. But as of this writing, GID may be medicalizing prehomosexual behavior, and thus contributing to the potential remedicalization of homosexuality.

On a more speculative note, we could consider changes within the context of a shift of psychiatric ideology from psychotherapeutic to pharmacological treatments and the growth of an expansive pharmaceutical industry (Conrad and Leiter, 2004). It is not beyond the realm of possibility that the pharmaceutical industry could develop some type of hormone therapy that allegedly could "treat" a deficient sexual orientation. But even if such an intervention were produced and promoted, for treatments to become legitimated would still require an accepted diagnosis (such as a more specific version of GID) and government-approved treatment of that "disorder."

The Emergence of HIV/AIDS

AIDS emerged as a deadly illness among gay men in the early 1980s. By the end of the decade AIDS had transformed gay communities; gay men were not only disproportionately contracting and dying from the disease, but gay communities became the center of AIDS activism and research.

Some social scientists have suggested that AIDS remedicalized homosexuality. Philip Kayal argues that "the present situation of gay AIDS is akin to previous 'medicalization of homosexuality' wherein gays are defined as both biologically and psychologically sick" (1993: 197). Sociologist Steven Epstein claims that because gay men were some of the first individuals to contract AIDS, the illness was framed as a "gay disease" among both public health workers and most Americans generally (Epstein, 1988). According to Epstein, being gay was perceived within popular culture as a "symptom" of AIDS. He argues that the medical communities' treatment of AIDS was a legacy of the medicalization of homosexuality within the psychiatric community. Epstein emphasizes, however, that AIDS differed from earlier perceptions of homosexuality in that not only the gay identity but the "gay community" and so-called gay lifestyle were medicalized (pp. 4, 13). Gregory Herek and John Capitanio similarly suggest that AIDS "repathologized" homosexuality in the mind of the average American. In a 1997 survey, the authors found that 40 percent of heterosexual respondents believe that gay sex, even among healthy gay men, was likely to result in the transmission of AIDS (1999: 1137). Dion Dennis refers to the "remedicalization of homosexuals in the wake of AIDS" (1997: 169).

For the most part, however, these authors use the term "medicalization" in a general way, rather than claiming that homosexuality itself had become a medical diagnosis again. In this section I briefly review the medical and public response to HIV/AIDS and its potential impact on the remedicalization of homosexuality.

The first conception and medical name of AIDS was "gay-related immune disorder" (GRID). The initial medical publications pointed out that because the patients were all homosexuals, there was some close association with homosexual lifestyle or sexual conduct (Shilts, 1987: 66–67; Epstein, 1996: 45–46). Evidence of AIDS in heterosexual populations was routinely ignored in this early period; researchers instead focused attention on the gay connection to the disease (Kayal, 1993; Epstein, 1996; S. Murray, 1996). Social scientists like Epstein and Kayal suggest that scientists and physicians constructed AIDS as a "gay disease" because they perceived the "homosexual lifestyle" of the 1970s as unhealthy. The early medical articles about AIDS cited 1970s articles that associated venereal disease and homosexuality. They came to see male homosexuality as a "medically problematic" situation (Epstein, 1988: 4).

In the early 1980s, AIDS was understood by the medical community through two frames, both of which promoted a view of AIDS as a "gay disease." The first frame, immune overload, saw AIDS as caused by immune deficiencies resulting from gay men's perceived excessive lifestyle (especially anal sex, multiple partners, and drug use). This perspective had huge public health implications. Any aspect of gay men's lives could be targeted for reform under the guise of disease prevention: choice of sex partner, number of sexual acts, drug use, attendance at bathhouses, and so on (Escoffier, 1998–99: 13).

The second medical frame focused on the spread of disease through specific risk groups. This model emerged with the recognition that AIDS was not isolated to gay men but was also common among intravenous drug users, hemophiliacs, and, in the first depictions, Haitians (Conrad, 1986). Homosexual behavior continued to be a target for the medical gaze and potential medical surveillance. With the discovery of the viral transmission of the disease, however, AIDS became associated more with specific behavior than with a particular group (Epstein, 1988: 25–26; see also Escoffier, 1998–99).

In this early period of HIV/AIDS, the medical community to a degree medicalized gay men's behavior in its conceptions of AIDS. While this framing of the disease did not last long, it resulted in an association of "homosexual lifestyle" and illness in the minds of many Americans. The media portrayed AIDS as a "gay disease," and the religious right presented gays and lesbians as a public health threat (Shilts, 1987). For example, the cover of a 1983 issue of *Moral Majority Report* included a picture of a family wearing surgical masks and the banner, "AIDS: Homosexual Disease Threatens American Families" (Bayer, 1985: 588).

The gay community was ambivalent about the framing of AIDS as a "gay disease" (Epstein, 1996: 53). Alarmed by the deaths in their community, gay activists were among the first and most persistent advocates drawing attention to the AIDS epidemic, creating support groups, and lobbying for AIDS research. According to Stephen Murray, gay men were more likely than the medical community to use terms such as "gay cancer" or "GRID" in early publications (1996: 104). The gay community, however, did not wholeheartedly accept the relationship between AIDS and homosexuality. For example, Randy Shilts notes that in 1982 the New York organization Gay Men's Health Crisis had over three hundred volunteers from the gay community but little support from gay leaders (1987: 180). Many gay men were also concerned that AIDS public health rhetoric was more a conservative strategy to restrain gay men's sexual expression (the sexual liberation they had fought for in the 1970s) than to protect their health. According to Shilts, it was not until the publication of an article entitled "1,112 and Counting," by Larry Kramer, in the *New York Native* in 1983 that the gay community in New York City rallied en masse around the issue of AIDS. By the late 1980s, however, AIDS had become a central gay cause, with organizations rallying support for those with the disease and AIDS research, which reinforced the notion of AIDS as largely a "gay disease" (Kayal, 1993: 3).

While the gay activism of the 1970s may have reduced the stigma of homosexuality, the emergence of AIDS renewed it. With its image as a disease related to a fast-track gay male lifestyle, AIDS tapped into a reservoir of existing fear of homosexuals (Conrad, 1986: 54). The new stigma, now due to alleged health reasons, led to discrimination in employment, medical care, insurance, and schools. Although the most overt AIDS-related discrimination had abated by the late 1980s, fears of contagion reinforced the stigmatizing link between AIDS and homosexuality.

Because of the perceived connection with homosexuality, the medical response to AIDS has been twofold: it includes both medical neglect and medical surveillance of gay men's behavior. Through lack of government funding and research, AIDS remained a largely misunderstood illness in the first half of the 1980s; this misunderstanding resulted in the deaths of thousands and the needless infection of countless others. Steven Epstein (1996) points out that leading gay activists were at the forefront in pressuring the government, scientists, and physicians to develop and deploy new treatments for AIDS.

On the other hand, the perceived association of AIDS and homosexuality resulted in the increased medical surveillance of gay men. This surveillance resulted in the closure of bathhouses, societal concerns about the quality of blood donations from gay individuals, debates about mandatory HIV testing, and the distribution of safe-sex guidelines within gay communities and more broadly (Shilts, 1987).

While the gay community wanted more medical research and treatment for people with AIDS, there were strong differences about how to regulate gay men's sexual activity as a means of preventing the spread of the disease. In particular, there were concerns within the gay community about medical surveillance of gay behavior and subsequent discrimination against those who tested positive for HIV. Congressional bills prohibited discrimination against individuals with HIV or AIDS, but confidentiality of HIV test results has never been completely assured by government proposals (Kayal, 1993: 88).

AIDS increased the medical surveillance of gay behavior and promoted the renewed stigmatization of homosexuality but did not medicalize homosexuality more generally. This was in large part due the strength of gay activism. Gay activists exposed the medical neglect of AIDS in the early years of the epidemic, pressed for research on the treatment of AIDS, demanded the distribution of AIDS treatments currently available, and provided the hospice services that hospitals were unwilling or unable to provide. By becoming "insiders" within the medical establishment, gay activists could both prevent the medical neglect of gay AIDS patients and ensure that medical treatment did not result in overt civil rights violations. Epstein argues there was an "expertification" of leading gay activists who instructed themselves in scientific methods and language in order to relay the concerns of the gay community to medical authorities (1996: 32–33). Ultimately, AIDS activism created a more cooperative relationship between physicians and AIDS patients (p. 346). Such cooperation resulted in safe-sex guidelines that were more gay-friendly (i.e., respecting sexual freedom) and in the gay community instructing medical practitioners about gay sexual practices (Escoffier, 1998–99: 2–9).

Genetics and Homosexuality

With a few notable exceptions (e.g., the repudiated work of Franz Kallman, 1952), from the 1930s through the 1980s there was little interest in or research on the hereditary or genetic origins of homosexuality. This was at least in part due to the disillusionment of scientists and the public with behavior genetics after the demise of eugenics (Paul, 1995), the lack of credible research evidence, and the horrors of the Holocaust. Biological theories fell out of favor both with the psychoanalysts who advocated the disease model and with gay activists who championed the "lifestyle" approach.

In the 1980s Richard Pillard and various colleagues published a few studies suggesting a possible genetic component to homosexuality (e.g., Pillard and Weinrich, 1986), but his studies received limited public exposure. In the 1990s, in the shadow of the Human Genome Project, there was an upsurge in research connecting homosexuality to genetics (Conrad and Markens, 2001). While these studies were not directly related to the genome project, the scientific and cultural climate had become much more open to genetic explanations of behavior, including homosexuality (Conrad, 1997).

Biological explanations of homosexuality emerged full force in the early 1990s. In 1991 the neuroscientist Simon LeVay published an article in the prestigious journal *Science* reporting a smaller hypothalamus in the brains of presumably gay men who had died from AIDS than in a comparison group (LeVay, 1991). This finding suggested that gay men may have a different biophysiology than heterosexual men. What the news media called "the gay brain" hypothetically could be of genetic origin. Despite some scientific critiques of this research, LeVay's findings were front-page news in a wide range of newspapers and news magazines (Conrad and Markens, 2001). That same year, Michael Bailey and Richard Pillard (1991) reported in the *Archives of General Psychiatry* that among identical twins, when one brother identified himself as homosexual, in 52 percent of the cases the twin did as well. The concordance was 22 percent for fraternal twins and 11 percent for siblings raised as brothers through adoption. The notion here was the more likely both twins were to be homosexual, the stronger the genetic connection. Although there were some criticisms of the study (e.g., there was no independent measure of homosexuality, and the data were collected via selective sampling through ads in gay periodicals), the news media amplified the findings with headlines like "New Study of Twins Finds Genetic Basis for Homosexuality" (*Boston Globe*, December 15, 1991) or "Genes Linked to Being Gay" (*USA Today*, December 17, 1991). While Bailey and Pillard's study showed at best some possible hereditary factors related to (male) homosexuality, it, along with LeVay's study and a few others (Allen and Gorski, 1992; Bailey et al., 1993), reopened the public discourse on the genetics of homosexuality.

The most prominent and, from a scientific point of view, sophisticated study of the genetics of homosexuality was published by Dean Hamer and his associates on

July 16, 1993, in the journal *Science*. The article reported the discovery of a genetic marker for homosexuality on the Xq28 region of the X chromosome (Hamer et al., 1993). Beginning that day, headlines around the world reported this discovery, which would soon be termed the "gay gene" (Conrad and Markens, 2001). Although Hamer and his associates published a second study in 1995 in *Nature Genetics* (Hu et al., 1995) with similar findings in a different sample, the research has not been replicated. Another research team attempted to replicate the findings and could not, yet they still maintained that there are genes for homosexuality, just not the ones Hamer found (Rice et al., 1999). Hamer has been a publicist for the genetic position. He published a popular book on his research, *The Science of Sexual Desire* (1994). He has also been quoted widely in the press and has appeared on dozens of radio and television programs. Even though, at best, what has been found is a genetic marker, not a gene, and there is yet to be replication of this research, the "gay gene" has become part of the common discourse in and outside of the gay and lesbian community.

Although the "gay gene" is a scientifically tentative notion, it has achieved broad public dissemination. Should a valid and verifiable gene or genes for sexual orientation be identified, there might be considerable pressure in some quarters for genetic testing, which could engender increased medicalization of homosexuality. Such testing might lead to the termination of pregnancies or, if ever available, genetic therapies for the "disorder."

The Gay Community and Perceptions of "Sexual Orientation"

In the late 1960s and 1970s, the gay liberation movement openly critiqued biological theories of sexuality. Writings by lesbian-feminists and gay activists stressed that sexuality was socially and not biologically constructed. The argument was that sexuality would be more fluid and diverse if heterosexuality were not mandated by society (Terry, 1999: 373; D'Emilio, 2002: 155). In a well-known article Adrienne Rich (1980) claimed, for example, that culturally ascribed "compulsory heterosexuality" makes women reluctant to explore sexual and emotional relationships with other women. To denote the fluidity in sexuality, activists generally referred to homosexuality as a "sexual preference."

By the 1980s, however, the gay community increasingly referred to homosexuality as an "orientation." The term "sexual orientation" implied that homosexuality was not a choice but an immutable part of one's personality. Especially within the male gay community, the concepts of "sexual orientation" and "sexual identity" became dominant. As historian John D'Emilio points out, "Identity spoke to something deep inside the individual, something that went to the very core of who one was" (2002: 157).

It was not until the 1990s that biological explanations of homosexuality became common. The "born-gay" philosophy became fashionable within gay and lesbian communities (Terry, 1999: 378; D'Emilio, 2002). A poll conducted by the *Advocate* found that nine of ten gay men believed they had been born gay (Kutchins and Kirk, 1997: 96). Indeed, biological explanations of homosexuality are commonly supported, not only among gays and lesbians but in American society as a whole. A Gallup poll from June 2001 asked Americans, "In your view, is homosexuality something a person is born with or is homosexuality due to other factors such as upbringing or environment?" Forty percent of respondents claimed that homosexuality was something one was born with, while only 39 percent emphasized environmental factors. This is a striking change from 1977, when only 13 percent of respondents embraced the born-gay philosophy (Gallup Organization, 2001). Similar polls demonstrate that individuals who believe in the genetic or biological origins of homosexuality are also more likely to support gay civil rights (Nuffield Council on Bioethics, 2002: 99). D'Emilio contends that there was a "rush, on the part of almost everyone except the most extremely homophobic elements of our society, to embrace the 'born gay' view of sexual identity" (2002: 154).

The born-gay explanation became popular because it fits within the current rhetoric of gay identity politics. Within the U.S. justice system, to obtain legislation protecting "civil rights," oppressed groups must argue that their group status is permanent and unchangeable. Lawyers in gay civil rights cases thus argue that homosexuality is a "sexual orientation" (D'Emilio, 2002: 10–12; Stein, 1999: 287). Moreover, genetic explanations of homosexuality counter beliefs by the religious right (and psychiatrists such as Socarides) that homosexuality is a psychopathology that can be "treated" (D'Emilio, 2002). The conservative argument holds that gay men can be given therapy so as to become heterosexual (Kutchins and Kirk, 1997: 95). Some observers have suggested that gay scientists such as Hamer and LeVay researched the "gay gene" as a means to silence claims that homosexuality is treatable (e.g., Terry, 1999: 384).

Many gays and lesbians also support biological explanations of homosexuality for more personal reasons. To some, it is uncomfortable to think that they chose the oppression and ostracism that comes with being homosexual in our society (D'Emilio, 2002: 161). Moreover, gays and lesbians often report that they had always "felt" gay, even in their earliest memories (Savin-Williams, 2001; D'Emilio, 2002: 157; Swidey, 2005).

While the born-gay ideology is popular, the gay community is not unified in its approach to social activism or beliefs about the origins of homosexuality. Queer politics, in particular, argues against organizing primarily around a gay identity. According to Steven Seidman, the "normalization" of homosexuality in our culture has fractured some gay communities and made it possible for gays and lesbians to see their sexuality as only a piece of their identity. As such, queer politics strives to liberate all sexualities from social control and is not narrowly focused on homosexuality (2001: 321–27). The view in the movement argues against essentializing identity and directly opposes the born-gay approach. Moreover, it is unclear whether the born-gay philosophy suggests an acceptance of a genetic explanation of sexuality. In her research on scientists and lay people's ideas about the relationship between biology and sexuality, Sarah Wilcox (2001) found that a reductionist understanding of biology as the determination of a dichotomous trait conflicted with the perspective of those associated with GLBT communities, who viewed sexuality in terms of a more multifaceted spectrum of variability. One response to this conflict was to view sexuality as innate yet involving spiritual, emotional, and psychological components not encompassed by either biology or a dichotomy between homosexuality and heterosexuality (Wilcox, personal communication).

The gay community expresses diversity in its responses to scientific studies of the "gay gene." The gay press was more ambivalent about the reports of the "gay gene" than the mainstream U.S. press. While the American mainstream press was generally optimistic about the supposed discovery of such a gene and relatively accepting of the scientific findings, the gay press was a bit more skeptical. Many articles stressed that evidence of a "gay gene" could support gay civil rights, but others voiced concerns about the possibility of prenatal testing and termination of pregnancies with a "gay fetus," as well as increased discrimination by insurance companies, employers, and the military (Conrad and Markens, 2001).

Ultimately, however, the affirmation of a "gay identity" or a "gay gene" by the gay community has altered how the medical establishment understands and treats gay, lesbian, bisexual, and transsexual individuals. In the 1980s, women and minorities chastised the medical community for underrepresenting minority populations in biomedical research and for assuming that the medical and health concerns of white males were the same for other populations. In the 1990s, the GLBT community entered the debate. They argued that gay, lesbian, bisexual, and transsexual individuals are also understudied and have unique health issues that are not reflected in the heterosexual population. The GLBT community pressured the medical establishment to recognize sexual "identity" as a variable affecting health status

(Epstein, 2003). As a result, "sexual orientation" has been included as an important demographic variable in the U.S. Department of Health and Human Services' "prevention agenda for the Nation," known as *Healthy People 2010* (2003: 131–32). Epstein argues that such a state-centered approach may open the door for the remedicalization of homosexuality: "The reification of identity tends to support the idea that certain groups either are susceptible to illness as a result of biological differences, or are prone to illness as a result of 'bad habits' and customs that are intrinsic to the group" (2003: 161).

AFTER DEMEDICALIZATION

Although the general trend over the past one hundred years has been toward medicalizing human problems, there are a small number of cases of demedicalization. Homosexuality remains the exemplary contemporary case of nearly complete demedicalization. Each of the four arenas I examined could compromise demedicalization or move toward the remedicalization of homosexuality.

The transformations in psychiatry are mixed. The centerpiece of demedicalization is the American Psychiatric Association's 1974 decision to remove homosexuality as a diagnosis from the DSM-II. For the most part this demedicalization has endured; the abolition of "ego-dystonic homosexuality" diagnosis surely strengthens demedicalization. On the other hand, writers have argued that the emergence of "gender identity disorder" medicalizes childhood gender deviance and thus potentially remedicalizes homosexuality. Gay, lesbian, bisexual, and transgender organizations walk a tightrope in supporting the GID diagnosis (presumably to allow transgendered individuals to have expensive sex-change operations covered by health insurance), because medicalizing childhood "prehomosexual behavior" could theoretically shift the balance toward a remedicalization of homosexuality. The National Association for Research and Therapy of Homosexuality is an Internet presence but a marginal player in terms of redefining homosexuality.

While several analysts suggested in the 1980s that the treatment and prevention of HIV/AIDS was engendering a remedicalization of homosexuality, two decades later this doesn't appear to be the case. The social response to HIV/AIDS has increased the stigmatization of homosexuality and medical surveillance of gay men's lives, but it has not contributed significantly to a remedicalization of homosexuality.

The renewed interest in genetics and Dean Hamer's discovery of what has been called a "gay gene" reflect a growing belief in and out of the gay community that people may be "born gay." While the scientific evidence is contentious, there is a widespread conception in the gay community that homosexuality is a sexual orien-

tation rather than a sexual preference. The response among gay activists to the geneticization of homosexuality, however, is mixed. Some see the genetic hypothesis
as evidence that homosexuality is natural, and thus it undermines claims that homosexuality is treatable. Others fear that it is a step in the direction of genetic therapy, remedicalization, and even genocide of potentially gay fetuses. What is apparent here is that it is not the genetic findings that are significant for medicalization,
but how they are interpreted. For example, arguments are made on both sides that
the discovery of a "gay gene" could be key in maintaining demedicalization or in
engendering a new remedicalization. It is not the scientific evidence itself that will
settle the issue, but rather what people do with it.

Overall, the nexus of medicalization potential seems to have shifted from psychiatry to genetics. Despite the murmurings around GID, psychiatry is unlikely to
resurrect medicalized psychiatric diagnoses or treatments. There is little interest in
homosexuality within the profession, especially as the dominant psychiatric treatment has shifted from psychotherapy to psychopharmacology. Although an increasing number of life problems have entered psychiatric jurisdiction in the past three
decades (Horwitz, 2002), the demedicalization of homosexuality remains stable.
The rise of the genetic paradigm and the enormous research apparatus it has
spawned make it likely that small genetic differences will be defined as evidence of
biomedical disorders (Conrad, 1997). While the current data remain contested and
limited, the publicity accorded to such findings highlights the power of the genetic
perspective.

Thirty years after the APA vote to eliminate the homosexuality diagnosis from the
DSM, homosexuality has been demedicalized but not vindicated. It remains subject
to stigma, and contentious issues like gay marriage, military service, and discrimination persist. Because the politicization of homosexual conduct underlay its demedicalization, it would likely take some kind of political upheaval to change it. Demedicalization can always be challenged, but it shows no real erosion at the moment.
Remedicalization seems unlikely, but as the political climate changes, so could homosexuality's place on the continuum from medicalization to demedicalization.

PART THREE

Constraints and Consequences

CHAPTER SIX

Measuring Medicalization

Categories, Numbers, and Treatment

Since the early 1970s, when sociologists began to write about medicalization, they have always claimed that it is increasing. While this appears to be a common-sense conclusion, it is fair to ask, What evidence has been presented to support this claim? In the 1980s at least one reviewer (Joffe, 1982) contended that the medicalization of deviance had peaked and was now decreasing in the wake of conservative social policy making. However, this frankly does not seem to be the case.

It would be difficult to quantify all trends in medicalization, because neither researchers nor government agencies tend to collect data with that question in mind. Yet if we are going to make claims about the increasing medicalization of society, it is ultimately incumbent on us to at least attempt to quantify the claim. This chapter presents a few specific cases that allow us to both examine some quantitative measures of medicalization and draw some inferences. Before I turn to these cases, I want to say something about the kinds of evidence usually presented to support the claim of increasing medicalization.

THE PROLIFERATION OF MEDICAL CATEGORIES FOR HUMAN PROBLEMS

Most often when sociologists write about the expansion of medical jurisdiction and the medicalization of life, they are referring to the increase in medicalized categories and diagnoses. For example, as pointed out in *Deviance and Medicalization* (Conrad and Schneider, 1980) and other publications in the 1980s (e.g., Wertz and Wertz, 1989), certain problems and conditions moved into the medical sphere during the previous century. These problems include mental illness, alcoholism, opiate

TABLE 6.1

Number of Diagnoses and Total Pages in DSM Versions I–IV, 1952–1994

Version	Year	Total Number of Diagnoses	Total Number of Pages
I	1952	106	130
I	1968	182	134
III	1980	265	494
III-R	1987	292	567
IV	1994	297	886

Source: American Psychiatric Association, *Diagnostic and Statistical Manual of Mental Disorders*, I-IV (Washington, D.C.: APA, 1952, 198, 1980, 1987, 1994). From Mayers and Horwitz, 2005.

addiction, childbirth, child abuse, and hyperactivity in children. Moreover, before the 1960s, categories such as attention-deficit/hyperactivity disorder (ADHD), post-traumatic stress disorder (PTSD), anorexia, fibromyalgia, premenstrual syndrome (PMS), and Alzheimer disease were either esoteric diagnoses or not yet described in the medical literature. Another measure of the growth of categories is the increase in the number of diagnoses in the *Diagnostic and Statistical Manual* from 106 in the original 1952 edition to nearly 300 disorders in the DSM-IV, which was published in 1994 (Mayes and Horwitz, 2005) (table 6.1).

As Stuart Kirk recently pointed out, the number of new disorders described in the various editions of the DSM in the past quarter-century keeps increasing:

> Since 1979, for example, some of the new disorders and categories that have been added include panic disorder, generalized anxiety disorder, post-traumatic stress disorder, social phobia, borderline personality disorder, gender identity disorder, tobacco dependence disorder, eating disorders, conduct disorder, oppositional defiant disorder, identity disorder, acute stress disorder, sleep disorders, nightmare disorder, rumination disorder, inhibited sexual desire disorders, premature ejaculation disorder, male erectile disorder and female sexual arousal disorder. If you don't see yourself on that list, don't fret, more are in the works for the next edition of the DSM. [2005: 5]

While some of these diagnoses (e.g., rumination disorder) are rather esoteric, others (panic disorder, post-traumatic stress disorder, social phobia, male erectile dysfunction) are so common as to be taken for granted as existing medical disorders.

In addition to the proliferation of medical categories and diagnoses, existing categories have also expanded. As chapter 3 points out, in the 1970s, hyperactivity was a diagnosis exclusively for children; by the 1990s, doctors were also identifying adult ADHD as the age criterion of the problem expanded. We can see a similar expansion in Alzheimer disease. When age was removed as a criterion for a diagnosis, more cases of senile dementia among the elder population were diagnosed as Alzheimer's (P. Fox, 1989). PTSD had its origin in Vietnam veterans who returned to the United States with a particular set of symptoms, including "flashbacks," insomnia, and intense anxiety. But in subsequent years PTSD has expanded to include survivors of sexual abuse, rape, violence, or natural disasters, and even people who have witnessed violence or disaster (W. Scott, 1990; Young, 1995). The medicalization of alcoholism, especially as defined by Alcoholics Anonymous, has expanded to include adult children of alcoholics, enablers, and especially codependents (L. Irvine, 1999). When Viagra was first introduced, it was marketed for people with erectile dysfunction due to aging, diabetes, or prostate surgery; in subsequent years, as noted in chapter 2, the notion of what constitutes erectile dysfunction has grown to include any possible concerns about sexual success (Conrad and Leiter, 1994). In other words, when one medicalized category gains legitimacy for a specific problem, it can be extended to include a wider array of similar, related, or analogous problems.

Sometimes broad general categories such as obesity and aging become medicalized. Obesity has always been a social and personal problem. Regimens for weight loss and diets have existed for centuries (H. Schwartz, 1986). In the United States, the incidence of obesity has risen so much that it has been called an epidemic. In the past two decades, at least, we have seen the medicalization of obesity; that is, obesity is viewed not just as a risk factor for medical problems like hypertension, heart disease, or diabetes, but as a disease in itself (Sobal and Maurer, 1995). In the 1970s, bariatric physicians (who specialize in obesity) composed an esoteric and perhaps even stigmatized specialty. Today gastric bypass operations are increasingly common for the extreme symptoms of obesity (morbid overweight). According to the American Society of Bariatric Surgery, in 2003, patients and their insurers spent more the $3.5 billion on 145,000 gastric bypass and similar operations (Freudenheim, 2005). The Centers for Disease Control announced in 2005 that obesity is the fastest growing health threat in the United States and will soon pass smoking as the number one risk factor for disease. Further research led the CDC to lower the number of deaths attributed to obesity, but it declared that obesity was still an epidemic (Zwillich, 2005). In 2004, Medicare revised its longstanding policy and removed the language that had said obesity was not an illness (http://usgovinfo.about.com/od/olderamericans/a/obesitypolicy.htm). By implicitly supporting the notion that obesity is a disease, the U.S. Department of Health and Human Services has provided an official imprimatur to the disease category and has opened the door for Medicare to cover the disorder as a medical problem.

Another broad category of increased medicalization is aging. Several researchers (e.g., Estes and Binney, 1989; Zola, 1991; S. Kaufman et al., 2004) have commented on this trend, which is manifested not only in the more frequent diagnosis of Alzheimer disease but also in the increasing medical jurisdiction over the whole process of aging—from minor memory deficits to mobility limits to the process of dying. Furthermore, while elders, in contrast to younger adults, have long taken a disproportionate amount of medication, the use of psychotropic medications has increased among the population over age 65 (Aparasu et al., 2001).

We can also look at the proliferation of categories that are medicalized in terms of gender. Both feminists and sociologists have long argued that women are more susceptible than men to medicalization, and more issues related to women—including childbirth, menstruation, birth control, fertility, PMS, pregnancy, and menopause—have been medicalized (Riessman, 1983; Riska, 2003). As demonstrated in chapter 2, however, in the past decade an increasing number of male life problems, including erectile dysfunction, baldness, and andropause, have been considered medical and have been addressed with medical treatments.

On the other side, how much demedicalization has occurred in the past century, and how much in the past thirty years? As in any dynamic social process, there have of course been cases where medical definitions or treatment are no longer deemed appropriate for a particular behavior or condition. Demedicalization occurs when a problem is no longer defined as medical, and medical treatments are no longer deemed appropriate. Obvious examples include masturbation, which in the late nineteenth century was deemed a disease and was often treated with radical medical interventions (Engelhardt, 1974) but is no longer considered to be a medical disorder or a sign of medical abnormality. The classic case of demedicalization in contemporary society is homosexuality. As pointed out in chapter 5, homosexuality was demedicalized in the 1970s, and despite changes in knowledge and in the political and social climate, it remains demedicalized. The other example that is sometimes raised is childbirth. Typical middle-class childbirth has changed since the 1950s, when a woman was alone with physicians and assistants in the delivery room, in stirrups, shaved and with an episiotomy, and often not even conscious while the doctor delivered the baby. Today, for nonrisky births it is much more typical for a woman to give birth in a birthing room, with her partner present, attended by a midwife or physicians. Often she is taking no medications. Soft music may be playing, and perhaps a friend is taking photographs. A fetal monitor of some type may be part of this serene scene. While this scenario is certainly a reformed version of the doctor-centered birthing of the 1950s, it is not demedicalized. To be demedicalized, the birth would take place at home, with a lay attendant, and without medical monitoring. Such births do occur, but they are rare; most births are still medical events, if more humane and interactive ones than five decades ago. Thus, in terms of categories, one would say that both pregnancy and childbirth are medicalized in our society.

In short, in terms of increased categories and expanded medical jurisdiction, medicalization has increased over the past century and perhaps most especially over the past three decades. But that being said, we still know little about how medicalization has grown, whether medicalization has increased in some areas and decreased in others, or how we might measure the extent of medicalization in a quantitative way. With the three cases I present in this chapter, I want take a few steps in this undertaking.

RISK SCARES AND MEDICALIZATION
Hormone Replacement Therapy

The medicalization of menopause has been well documented in the sociological literature (McCrea, 1983; Bell, 1987; Lock, 1993).[1] The current medical conception of menopause has its roots in the 1930s, with the publication of a number of medical articles and the development of both natural and synthetic estrogens (Bell, 1987). Some analysts suggest that menopause became medicalized because of medical claims that the "symptoms" of menopause were a sign of a disease, while others contend that it was because of the availability of a treatment. Both were probably important, as numerous articles were written in the medical literature about the disease qualities of menopause, but clearly the introduction of hormone replacement therapy (HRT) was key in the popularization of the medical conception and treatment.[2]

The early medical reports suggested that estrogen could reduce menopausal symptoms, and there were numerous claims of the benefits of the drug for the "hormone-deficiency disease" of menopause. Medical articles claimed that estrogen "prevented breast and genital cancer and other problems of aging" (McCrea, 1983: 112). Estrogen was touted as a treatment not only for menopausal symptoms but also for the deterioration of old age. Robert Wilson's book *Feminine Forever* claimed that hormone medications would combat the disease of menopause with estrogen replacement therapy (ERT) and women would be saved from "being condemned to witness the death of their womanhood" (quoted in McCrea, 1983: 113). The idea that menopausal women had an estrogen deficiency became common medical knowledge, and women were encouraged to take estrogen replacement therapy. By 1975, estrogen was the fifth most frequently prescribed drug in the United States (McCrea, 1983), with more than 30 million prescriptions written a year (Hersh et al., 2004).

From the beginning, there were concerns about adverse effects from ERT, including increased rates of endometrial cancer (McCrea, 1983). The National Institute of Aging concluded in 1979, "ERT is only effective in the treatment of hot flashes and vaginal atrophy, and if used at all, should be administered on a cyclical basis (three weeks of estrogen, one week off) at the lowest dose for the shortest possible time" (McCrea, 1983: 115). The prescriptions dropped from an estimated 30 million in 1975 to 15 million five years later (Hersh et al., 2004).

When a "safer" alternative, a convenient combination of estrogen and progestin, appeared in the 1980s, prescriptions for HRT increased. In addition to the safer drug, studies in the 1980s seemed to show that HRT was effective in reducing the impact of osteoporosis and the risks of coronary artery disease. In the 1980s, pharmaceutical companies widely promoted HRT as a way to prevent such ravages of aging as osteoporosis (Worcester and Whatley, 1992). In 1992 the American College of Physicians recommended that "most menopausal women should take HRT unless they were already at high risk for breast cancer" (Cowley and Springen, 2002: 38). Based on a meta-analysis, experts in 1999 stated that "almost all menopausal women will benefit from HRT, especially those with risk factors for coronary heart disease" (Keating et al., 1999: 545). Prempro, a convenient combination that could be taken as a single pill daily, was introduced in 1995. Pharmaceutical companies heavily promoted HRT; usage of HRT increased from 17 percent of women over age 50 in 1992 to 33 percent in 2001. By the mid-1990s in the United States, nearly half of all postmenopausal women were prescribed long-term HRT. In 1999 more than 15 million women in the United States were taking HRT; these numbers remained stable until 2002 (Hersh et al., 2004).

In July 2002 an article in the *Journal of the American Medical Association* reported that an important HRT study, the Women's Health Initiative (WHI), had been terminated in light of findings about the risks of the drug. The study, supported by the National Institutes of Health (NIH), compared outcomes of 16,600 women randomized to receive HRT with estrogen and progestin verses placebo. Although it was scheduled as an eight-year clinical trial, this part of the study was ended after just over five years because the investigators discovered that the cumulative risks of severe adverse outcomes, including breast cancer, coronary heart disease, venous thromboembolisms (blood clots), and strokes, outweighed the benefits of reduced osteoporosis and colon cancer. Results of another study, the Heart and Estrogen/ Progestin Replacement Study (HERS II), were published in *JAMA* at the same time. This study found that after 6.8 years, hormone therapy did not reduce the risk of cardiovascular events in women with coronary heart disease (Grady et al., 2002). Other reports suggested that HRT could actually increase the risk of Alzheimer disease and other dementias (Shumaker et al., 2002).

The results from the WHI study made headline news and created confusion and new fears among providers and patients alike. The Food and Drug Administration and major medical organizations (e.g., the North American Menopause Society, the American College of Obstetrics and Gynecology, and the American College of Physicians) all changed their position on HRT within a few months of the study's publication. Most stated that there was no role for HRT in disease prevention and that HRT should be used only to treat severe menopausal symptoms, and then only for short periods of time. They advised women who were taking HRT to consult their physicians and consider discontinuing the medication (Stephenson, 2003; North American Menopause Society, 2003).

In the first month after the WHI publication, more than four hundred related news articles and twenty-five hundred television and radio reports appeared (Schwartz and Woloshin, 2004). The news precipitated a massive discontinuance of HRT. A major national study reported a dramatic 43 percent decline in prescriptions of estrogen plus progestin eighteen months after the WHI results (Majumdar et al., 2004). Sales of Wyeth's estrogen-progestin combination Prempro plummeted 50 percent between 2002 and 2003 (S. Smith, 2003).

The original WHI study did not address quality-of-life issues. A 2003 *New England Journal of Medicine* article based on the WHI study showed that practically no differences existed between the HRT-treated and placebo groups on virtually all measures related to quality of life (Hays et al., 2003). In 2004 the National Institutes of Health suspended an HRT study that focused on estrogen only; it concluded that ERT slightly increased the risk of stroke and did not prevent heart disease (Writing Group for the Women's Health Initiative Investigators, 2004). Researchers were concluding that there was little value but considerable risk to long-term ERT therapy, and evidence suggested that HRT therapy was useful only on a short-term basis for women suffering from severe hot flashes and night sweats: "New guidelines recommend against routine hormone therapy for chronic conditions, and current users have been advised to taper doses toward discontinuation" (Hersh et al., 2004: 47).

I draw certain inferences from this case. First, the medicalization of menopause as a conception or diagnosis was related to the development of HRT treatment. Second, when HRT treatment became easier and safer, the prevalence of hormone treatment for menopausal women increased markedly. At one time half of all postmenopausal women were being treated with HRT. Because the onset of menopause triggered the treatment, one could say that this number likely approximated the actual number of women for whom menopause was medicalized. We don't know, however, how many women were taking hormone treatment for menopause per se and how many were taking it for wholly preventive purposes, nor do we know how many women were taking it for both reasons. However, my best approximation of the number of women whose menopause was medicalized with HRT is 15 million in 2002.

When the WHI and similar studies were published, HRT treatment plummeted. Did this mean that these women's menopause was demedicalized? This is an empirical question, and it requires the measurement of how many of these women and their doctors continued to define menopause as a disorder requiring medical treatment. My sense is that the HRT scare and reduction did not diminish the conceptual medicalization of menopause but only the number of women being treated for the condition of menopause.

Breast Implants

The case of breast implants provides an analogous situation. Breast implants are perhaps better seen as an example of enhancement than of medicalization, but they can also be seen as an example of medicalized enhancement. While only a few physicians saw small breasts as a disease ("micromastia"), both surgeons and women did see medical solutions to the "problem" of small breasts (Jacobson, 2000: 66). The ideal size of breasts varies by culture; this case represents the cultural view in the United States in the late twentieth century.

Until the 1950s there was only limited medical interest in enlarging small breasts. While there were some less than fully successful medical procedures to increase breast size before this time (see Conrad and Jacobson, 2003), the introduction of silicone breast implants in the 1960s initiated the modern era of breast augmentation. Early silicone injections proved to have serious problems, but women "continued to clamor for a solution to [small breasts] and surgeons continued to search for one" (Haiken, 1997: 255). Silicone implants were introduced by Dow Corning in 1962, and by 1970 the company had sold an estimated fifty thousand implants. These modest sales numbers grew. Between the early 1960s and 1990, approximately 2 million women received silicone implants (Yalom, 1997: 237; Jacobson, 2000). Of these cases, 20 percent were for reconstructive purposes following mastectomy, while 80 percent were for cosmetic purposes (Zimmerman, 1998).

But all was not well with silicone implants. Articles began to appear in the popular press and in academic journals questioning the safety of the implants and highlighting the problems, including silicone gel leakage, hardening of the breasts, carcinogenicity, and autoimmune disease. Throughout the 1990s, as the controversy publicly exploded, tens of thousands of women joined legal suits that resulted in several global settlements against implant manufacturers. In 1992 the FDA called for a voluntary moratorium on the distribution and implementation of the devices, to which the manufacturers agreed (see Conrad and Jacobson, 2003).

Directly following the peak of the controversy and the 1992 ban, breast implant procedures plummeted. In 1990, 120,000 implants were performed; in 1992, there were only 30,000 (Jacobson, 2000). However, with the introduction of "safer" saline breast implants, the numbers of breast implants increased by 92 percent over the next decade. This trend continues. According to the American Society for Aesthetic Plastic Surgery, in 2004 there were over 334,000 breast augmentations in the United States (ASAPS, 2004). This procedure is now the second most popular cosmetic surgery, following liposuction.

What is interesting here is both the widespread use of medicalized enhancements to change bodies and the trajectory of consumption. Cosmetic surgery has become far more popular and acceptable than it was several decades ago. This popularity is apparent in television shows like *Extreme Makeover* and *The Swan*, as well as in the profound increase in cosmetic surgical procedures (Sullivan, 2001). The statistic of 2 million breast implants over three decades (1960–90) seemed formidable, but the current rate of 340,000 a year in the United States is astounding. At this rate we can estimate more than 3 million breast enhancement procedures per decade. Overall, the number of cosmetic surgical interventions increased by 49 percent between 2003 and 2004. While thus far 90 percent of these were for women, the number of men is rapidly increasing as well (see ASAPS, 2005a). The huge expansion in cosmetic surgery makes it abundantly clear that medicalized solutions to problems of the body are increasingly common and accepted in our society.

The trajectory of demand for and use of breast implants is informative. Until the 1990s the number of breast implants was steadily rising, but after the controversy about the risks of silicone implants, the number of procedures dropped enormously. With the introduction of a safer alternative, saline implants, however, the numbers of implants escalated far beyond previous levels. What happened, of course, is that the demand for medical breast augmentations never changed; only the number of procedures did.

Perhaps the example of breast implants is instructive about the future of HRT. The use of HRT has fallen precipitously since 2002 in the wake of reports of its dangers. But if some safer alternative becomes available, it is likely that the HRT trajectory will come to look a great deal like that of breast implants: the numbers will rise, perhaps to higher levels than previously.

In both these examples we saw a precipitous drop in the use of medicalized solutions after the discovery and publicizing of the risks of these solutions to the putative problems. But did the actual medicalization of these entities change? I would argue that the medicalization itself—the defining of the problem in medical terms—did not change. What changed was the implementation of medicalized interventions. As noted in the example of breast enhancement, when apparently safer alternatives became available, the number of medicalized interventions rose rapidly. Neither the conception nor the demand had changed; the adverse effects and risks of the medical treatment or procedure had merely dampened the use of medical intervention.

We can measure two different aspects of medicalization: definition and implementation. It is difficult to put numbers on the breadth and depth of definitions; it is easier to measure use.

INCREASING PRESCRIPTIONS OF PSYCHOTROPIC MEDICATIONS FOR ADOLESCENTS

My interest in medicalization was first kindled in my research on ADHD in the early 1970s.[3] When I wrote about hyperactivity (as ADHD was commonly called), I would use existing studies of prevalence to indicate the number of children who were considered as having ADHD (all numbers here refer to the U.S. population, unless otherwise specified). The numbers that I cited were always from other sources, and they were estimates of the percentage of children who had ADHD, not measures of the numbers of children who were treated. The latter numbers simply did not exist, although I noted that the estimated prevalence of hyperkinesis was 3–10 percent of the elementary school population. In a footnote I observed that most estimates varied between 3 and 5 percent of the population, with an occasional estimate up to 20 percent. I also suggested in a footnote that "it is likely that between 250,000 and 500,000 children have been identified as hyperkinetic" (Conrad, 1976: 9). It was apparent to me then, as it is now, that these numbers were not based on much; rather, they were extrapolations from small community studies or best-judgment estimates.

In the 1970s it was common to use the estimate that 3–5 percent of school-aged children were hyperactive (i.e., had ADHD), with a 9 to 1 ratio of boys to girls. Current estimates vary, but generally they are larger: the CDC (2002) estimates that 7 percent of U.S. children aged 6–11 have ADHD; a national survey suggests that 4 million schoolchildren have ADHD (U.S. Department of Health and Human Services, 2004); and one expert claims that there are 8 million adults with ADHD (AMA Science News, 2004).

Treatment rates have increased as well. From 2000 to 2002, 5 million children aged 5–17 were treated for ADHD, up from 2.6 million in 1994–96 (U.S. Department of Health and Human Services, 2004: 62). Gender estimates have changed so that now boys are considered 3 to 1 more likely to have ADHD (Biederman et al., 1996). The diagnosis of ADHD remains twice as high among white children compared with black and Hispanic children (U.S. Department of Health and Human Services, 2004: 14). Using a different kind of measure, it has been estimated that there was a 700 percent increase in prescriptions of stimulant medications in the 1990s (Diller, 1997). There is no question that the number of children treated with stimulant medications for ADHD and related problems has increased markedly in three decades.

Thus, thirty years after my original study of hyperactive children was completed, we see a far more widespread use of psychotropic medications, including stimulants for ADHD. At least from the drug company's perspective, we can see Ritalin and the other stimulants for ADHD as pioneer drugs, as the first drugs widely marketed for children's behavioral, learning, and emotional problems. Since the 1970s there has been a notable upsurge in the number of drugs prescribed for children's behavior and the number of problems for which they are marketed.

By the 1990s it had become apparent both that the notion of ADHD had expanded (see chapter 3) and that the use of psychotropic medications for children and adolescents was increasing at a rapid rate. If one was interested in the medicalization of the behavior of children and adolescents, it would be necessary to look beyond ADHD and stimulants and be inclusive of other types of psychotropic medications.

In consort with three colleagues who had experience in drug and adolescent research as well as a greater understanding of quantitative measurement, I set out to examine the trends in the use of psychotropic medications among adolescents. It was clear to us at the outset, based on existing research, that prescriptions for psychotropics had increased through the early 1990s. However, no studies had focused primarily on adolescents. Based on our impressions from various sources, this seemed like a population for whom psychotropic prescribing was becoming particularly widespread, and no study had gone beyond 1997. I will briefly summarize our study here and indicate how it relates to measuring medicalization. For details on the study's method and findings, please see the original article (Thomas et al., 2006).

While stimulants like Ritalin and newer drugs like Concerta and Adderall had been approved for use with children, few of the widely used antidepressants, especially the selective serotonin reuptake inhibitors (SSRIs), had FDA approval for use with children under the age of 18. But physicians can prescribe such drugs, approved for adults, for children on an "off-label" basis. Since the 1980s there has been evidence of the increased use of both stimulants for ADHD (Olfson et al., 2003) and antidepressants (Zito et al., 2002) among youth. Although adolescents had relatively low prescription rates for psychotropic medications before the 1990s (Olfson et al.,

2002, 2003; Zito et al., 2003), several recent studies have noted that adolescents as an age group have one of the highest rates of increase in psychotropic use, particularly SSRIs (see Thomas et al., 2006). However, none of these prior studies measures the use of psychotropics after 1997, the year that the Food and Drug Administration Modernization Act and additional FDA directives were enacted. These directives allow for looser restrictions on off-label drug promotion and direct-to-consumer (DTC) advertising. In addition, several new psychotropic medications were introduced after 1996.

Our study used data from the National Ambulatory Medical Care Survey, or NAMCS, an annual, nationally representative sample of office-based physician visits by individuals who are insured and uninsured, to investigate the prescription rates for a range of psychotropic medications (stimulants, SSRIs, and other classes of psychotropic drugs). We examined trends in psychotropic prescribing rates for adolescents from 1994 to 2001.

Our analysis showed that office-based visits resulting in psychotropic prescriptions rose from 3.4 percent in 1994–95 to 8.3 percent in 2000–2001 (significance $p < .001$). This represented a 2.5-fold increase in eight years. Adjusting for population, this meant that the rate of physician visits resulting in adolescents receiving a psychotropic prescription increased from 52.2 per 1,000 to 141.8 per 1,000 in the same time period. In addition, the greatest growth was in the post-1999 period, when the rate of increase in psychotropic prescriptions nearly doubled. Interestingly, over the entire period roughly one-fifth of individuals who visited a physician and received a prescription for psychotropics had no mental health diagnosis. The increases were similar for both males and females and for both stimulants and antidepressants. For each time period, about one-third of the adolescents who visited a physician and received a prescription for a psychotropic medication had a diagnosis of ADHD. By 2001, one in every ten of all office visits to physicians by adolescent males (for whatever reason) resulted in the prescription of a psychotropic medication.

Our study illustrates several important points. First, it is sometimes important to go beyond specific diagnoses if we are to measure medicalization. One-third of those visits resulting in a psychotropic medication were for ADHD, but most were for other diagnoses (e.g., depression, affective psychoses, and "neurotic disorder"). One-fifth had no mental health diagnoses at all. Stimulants such as Ritalin are no longer the most common medications prescribed to children and adolescents.

Second, when one examines trends over time, interesting patterns may emerge. All previous studies in the past decade have shown increases in psychotropic prescribing to children (see also W. O. Cooper et al., 2006); this increase may be due to expanding definitions of psychiatric problems (Horwitz, 2002), the introduction of new medications with fewer apparent adverse effects, and a reduced threshold for prescribing psychotropics in this post-Prozac era. SSRIs and Ritalin treatment have become common and well accepted among physicians and the public alike. Our data show that there may be a significant rise after 1999. We speculate that this increase may be due to both the introduction of new medications in the period and the impact of DTC advertising. While our data can't directly examine the DTC pharmaceutical promotion or reduced threshold hypotheses, these may be important factors in spurring this large increase in psychotropic prescriptions, especially when other prescriptions, like antibiotics, are declining among children and adolescents.

Third, in recent years there has been concern about the overuse of psychotropics among children and adolescents and apprehension about the risks and potential adverse effects of these drugs (e.g., the adolescent suicide risk from SSRIs; concern about excess deaths with ADHD drugs) (Jureidini et al., 2004; Whittington et al., 2004; R. Rubin, 2006). These are further reasons to be concerned about the widespread medicalization of the problems of children and adolescents.

In this context, it is worth noting that there is some evidence of a 20 percent drop in SSRI use among children from March to December 2004 (Rosack, 2005). This is likely a result of the risk scare that SSRIs may increase suicidality in children and adolescents (Jureidini et al., 2004), which prompted the British medical authority to ban SSRIs for children and the FDA to add a "black box" warning to the drug labels. It is unclear, however, whether this decline in use will be just a blip in the continual rise of SSRI use with children and adolescents or if it will be a long-lasting trend. But as with other risk scares mentioned above, the decrease of medication use does not necessarily indicate that there has been any reduction in medicalization of children's problems.

Whatever the explanation, the 2.5-fold increase in visits that result in a prescription for a psychotropic medicine is at least some indirect measure of the increased medicalization of the social and emotional difficulties of adolescents. Problems that a decade or two ago would not have been deemed appropriate for medication are now managed with psychotropics, even apparently sometimes without any mental health diagnosis; this clearly indicates a greater implementation of medicalized solutions for human problems.

WILL HALF OF AMERICANS BECOME MENTALLY ILL?

During the summer when I was writing this chapter, I was startled by headlines like "Most Will Be Mentally Ill at Some Point, Study Says" (*San Francisco Chronicle*, June 7, 2005) or "Mental Illness Will Hit Half of U.S." (*New York Times*, June 7,

2005). Just as I was thinking about measures of medicalization, here were reports of studies suggesting that half of all Americans will become mentally ill. Were these the reports of a major epidemic or a further medicalization of life problems?[4]

These news stories reported findings from the 2001–3 National Comorbidity Survey (NCS-R), a once-a-decade study of the state of our country's mental health (Kessler et al., 2005a, 2005b, 2005c). The study is based on a national survey of more than 9,000 respondents aged 18–54. This survey replicates a similar survey completed a decade earlier, and the study presents findings on many aspects of mental health and its treatment. This is a commendable task, because mental illness in the community is notoriously difficult to measure. To its credit, this survey draws attention to the problems of mental illness, attempts to find mentally disordered people who are in the community but not being treated, and uses enormously sophisticated methods. This is a major study by any standard, and it has produced over a dozen articles already, many in the best medical journals. Surely more will come.

The authors present some stunning findings: Nearly half the population will have a diagnosable mental disorder (based on the diagnoses in the DSM-IV) in their lifetime. A large segment of the populace will at some time in their lives have anxiety disorders (28.8%), impulse control disorders such as attention deficit disorder (24.8%), and mood disorders (20.8%) (Kessler et al., 2005a). Twelve-month prevalence rates estimate that 26.2 percent will have some kind of DSM-IV disorder within a year (22.3% classified as serious, 37.3% as moderate, and 40.4% as mild) (Kessler et al., 2005b). The researchers also report that although the number of individuals being treated for a mental disorder has increased over the last ten years, most people who have a mental disorder still do not receive treatment (Kessler et al., 2005c).

In terms of medicalization, there are several ways to interpret these figures. First, it seems that a hugely wide range of behaviors must be included in this paradigm so that roughly *half* the population has a lifetime probability of mental disorder. Second, one wonders where the line between a mild disorder and normal life difficulties is drawn. Studies like these tend to pathologize difficulties as symptoms and create putative diagnoses. Third, while treatment of mental disorders has increased in the last decade, most individuals who have a putative mental disorder do not receive treatment. From a psychiatric viewpoint, this means there is a great deal of untreated morbidity; from a medicalization view, it means many people have problems that could be medicalized. While there are undoubtedly people with serious disorders who are untreated, just as likely there are people with mild problems who are diagnosed and treated, most likely with psychotropic medications. So what we have here is an expansion of what is seen as a potentially diagnosable mental disorder. Without being too cynical, one could say this study is a boon for the drug companies; consider the yet untapped market for their products.

Beyond medicalization, though, to assess these kinds of findings we need to ask where the numbers come from and whether they make sense from a clinical point of view. Allan Horwitz and Jerome Wakefield have been examining the sources of these types of community mental health surveys for some time (Horwitz, 2002; Horwitz and Wakefield, forthcoming). My analysis below draws heavily on their work.

No matter how sophisticated the methodology of the study, if its definitions of a mental disorder are faulty, the results will be questionable. The extraordinarily high prevalence rates of untreated mental disorders reported in community studies like the NCS-R inherently *overstate* the number of people with mental disorders. The inflated prevalence rates stem from the standardized and decontextualized questions about symptoms that do not distinguish normal experience of distress in response to negative life events from genuinely pathological conditions. Both are equally classified as signs of mental disorders. As Horwitz and Wakefield (forthcoming) note, because people who experience normal reactions to life events are less likely than people with serious disorders to seek medical attention, the process inflates estimates of untreated mental disorder.

Community psychiatric surveys like the NCS-R use questions that are virtually exact translations from those designated for diagnoses in the DSM. The DSM frequently requires a certain number of symptoms (e.g., difficulty sleeping, loss of appetite, fatigue, depressed mood, feeling worthless) to make a diagnosis (e.g., depression). But this manual is meant for clinical diagnoses, and the symptoms are seen as part of a patient history and in the context of their lives. For studies like the NCS-R, the DSM's symptoms are put into standardized, closed-ended questions about symptoms, and respondents are asked to report whether they have had any of these "symptoms" in the past two weeks. The research interview completely excludes any discussion of context or the individual's history. Thus, it is impossible to judge if a person has trouble sleeping, depressed mood, and fatigue because he or she has lost a job or a loved one or whether it is unrelated to life events. Unlike clinical interviews, the context of the individual's "symptoms" is completely excluded, which leads to a considerable overestimation of the amount of psychiatric pathology in the community. Such surveys conflate normal, transitory life distress with the potential for a serious mental disorder. Survey-driven diagnoses are not equivalent to the clinical diagnoses that can be provided by a psychiatrist. Many of the "symptoms" that are seen as part of a survey-rendered diagnosis would probably never be brought to the attention of a professional, and many are likely inconsequential and transitory.[5]

In short, only with the broadest definition could we expect half the population to have a diagnosable mental disorder in their lifetime. Community studies like the NCS-R inevitably overestimate the prevalence of mental disorders. They include problems that don't require professional treatment and pathologize normal life difficulties. This encourages the medicalization of everyday troubles and suggests psychiatric treatment as their solution. This approach aligns with, and perhaps encourages, the enormous rise over the past decade in the use of psychotropic medications for an increasing range of problems. Of course, some people who are severely distressed could benefit from professional treatment. But surveys like the NCS-R create overly expansive notions of mental disorders that inadvertently contribute to the increasing medicalization of life problems.

TREATMENT, MEASUREMENT, AND MEDICALIZATION

What can we conclude from our three examples of measuring medicalization? Clearly, by all standards, categories, treatment rates, and measures of pathology, medicalization is continuing to increase. The HRT/breast implant case suggests that although medicalization and medical treatments are intertwined, one doesn't necessarily affect the other. For example, a medicalized "treatment" may be curtailed by the discovery of its serious risks; however, when a "safer" alternative appears, medicalized solutions are again implemented, at the same rates as before or even more. Thus, the medicalization remained the same, only the implementation changed. The second example shows that increasing numbers of adolescent troubles are treated by psychotropic medications, both with and without a mental health diagnosis. What is interesting here is the steady escalation in treatment over the past fifteen years, apparently boosted by the advent of DTC advertising, which creates a greater demand for medical solutions to life problems. It will be interesting to see whether the current concerns with suicide risk among adolescents taking SSRIs or the recent reports of increased cardiac risks from stimulants (Nissan, 2006) will have an impact on the number of individuals who receive treatment with these drugs.

Finally, the National Comorbidity Study example illustrates how psychiatric research itself can potentially medicalize more of life's problems and overstate the existence of untreated psychiatric "pathology." Findings like this could spur an actual increase in medical treatments for minor life difficulties and serve as a rationale for extending psychotropic treatments to larger portions of the population. One might imagine new DTC ads heralding the huge amount of untreated mental disorders unearthed by the NCS-R and suggesting that if you have this "symptom," you should ask your doctor if (insert specific SSRI) is right for you. This scenario then becomes a medicalization-amplifying feedback loop.

CHAPTER SEVEN

The Shifting Engines of Medicalization

When I first began studying medicalization in the 1970s the most important forces behind medicalization were physicians, social movements and interest groups, and various organizational or interprofessional activities. But with the significant changes in medicine in the past three decades, there has also been a shift in the forces that underlie increasing medicalization. Some of this is already apparent from the cases examined in previous chapters, but in this chapter I want to identify and examine how three major changes in medical knowledge and organization have engendered a shift in the engines that drive medicalization in Western societies: biotechnology, consumers, and managed care.

BIOTECHNOLOGY

Various forms of biotechnology have long been associated with medicalization. Whether it be technology such as forceps for childbirth (Wertz and Wertz, 1989) or drugs for distractible children (Conrad, 1975), technology has often facilitated medicalization. These drugs or technologies were not the driving force in the medicalization process; facilitating, yes, but not primary. But this is changing. The pharmaceutical and biotechnology industries are becoming major players in medicalization.

The Pharmaceutical Industry

The pharmaceutical industry has long been involved in promoting its products for various ills. In the original edition of our book *Deviance and Medicalization* (Conrad and Schneider, 1980), the examples of Ritalin, methadone, and psychoactive medications were all a piece of the medicalization process. However, in each of these cases it was physicians and other professionals who were in the forefront. With Ritalin there were drug advertisements promoting the treatment of "hyperactivity" in children and no doubt "detailing" to doctors (e.g., drug company representatives' sales visits to doctors' offices). But it was the physicians who were at the center of the issue.

This has changed. While physicians are still the gatekeepers for many drugs, the pharmaceutical companies have become a major player in medicalization. In the post-Prozac world, the pharmaceutical industry has been more aggressively promoting its wares to physicians and especially to the public. Some of this is not new. For most of the twentieth century the industry has been limited to promoting its wares to physicians through detailing, sponsoring medical events, and advertising in professional journals. However, since the passage of the Food and Drug Administration Modernization Act of 1997 and subsequent directives, the situation has changed.

Revisions in FDA regulations allowed for a wider usage and promotion of off-label uses of drugs and facilitated direct-to-consumer (DTC) advertising, especially on television (see Conrad and Leiter, 2005). While part of the FDA rationale was that such advertising would be educational and "awareness raising" for the public, this change in regulation has altered the game for the pharmaceutical industry; companies can now advertise directly to the public and create markets for their products. Overall, pharmaceutical industry spending on television advertising increased sixfold between 1996 and 2000, to $2.5 billion (Rosenthal et al., 2002), and it has been rising steadily since; in 2004 the industry spent $4 billion on DTC advertising, the great bulk of it on television (Lenzer, 2005). Drug companies now spend nearly as much on DTC advertising as on advertising to physicians in medical journals, especially for "blockbuster drugs that are prescribed for common complaints such as allergy, heart burn, arthritis, 'erectile dysfunction,' depression and anxiety" (Relman and Angell, 2002: 36). A Kaiser Family Foundation study showed that from every $1 invested in DTC advertising, the companies obtained $4.20 in sales (Lenzer, 2005). A brief reprise of the cases of Paxil and Viagra can illustrate this, although there are many other examples (see Conrad and Leiter, 2004).

Male impotence was a medical problem long before the FDA approved Viagra as treatment for erectile dysfunction (ED) in 1998. As presented in chapter 2, a demand for treatments for erectile problems existed before Pfizer began advertising Viagra. When Viagra was first introduced, it was promoted as a treatment for older men with ED problems related to diabetes, prostate cancer, and other medical problems (Loe, 2001). Pfizer soon recognized that there was a larger market for the drug,

so began promoting ED as a common sexual difficulty and Viagra as the medical solution. Virtually any man might consider himself to have some type of erectile or
sexual dysfunction. "Ask your doctor if Viagra is right for you," the ads suggest.

Sales of Viagra were sensational. Viagra became a top-selling medication (see
chapter 2). By 2003, Levitra and Cialis had been introduced as improvements and
competitors for a share of this large market. The drug industry has expanded the notion of ED and has even subtly encouraged the use of Viagra-like drugs as an enhancement to sexual pleasure and relationships. Recent estimates suggest a potential market of more than 30 million men in the United States alone (Tuller, 2004).
The medicalization of ED and sexual performance has significantly increased in the
past six years and shows no signs of abating.

When Prozac was introduced in 1987, it was the first wave of new antidepressants
called selective serotonin reuptake inhibitors. SSRIs were as effective as older antidepressants or better, with fewer disturbing side effects. These drugs caused a bit of
a revolution in the pharmaceutical market (Healy, 1997), and with $10.9 billion in
sales in 2003 have become the third best selling class of drugs in the United States
(IMS Health, 2004). As noted in chapter 1, when Paxil (paroxetine hydrochloride)
was approved by the FDA in 1996, it joined a crowded market for antidepressants.
The manufacturer of Paxil, now called GlaxoSmithKline, sought FDA approval
to promote its product for the "anxiety market," especially social anxiety disorder
(SAD) and generalized anxiety disorder (GAD). In a sophisticated advertising campaign, SAD was promoted as a common mental health problem with Paxil as its
treatment. The marketing campaign for Paxil has been extremely successful. Paxil
became one of the three most widely recognized drugs, after Viagra and Claritin
(Marino, 2002) and in 2001 was ranked as the number nine prescription drug, with
U.S. sales of approximately $2.1 billion and global sales of $2.7 billion. By 2004,
Paxil's sales ranking had dropped considerably after some well-publicized reports
of adverse effects (see www.p-d-r.com/ranking/WoodMac_Top100.pdf). How much
Paxil was prescribed for SAD is impossible to discern, but by now both Paxil and
SAD are everyday terms. While there have been some concerns raised about Paxil
recently (Marshall, 2004), it is clear that GlaxoSmithKline's campaign for Paxil increased the medicalization of anxiety, implying that shyness and worrying may be
medical problems, with Paxil as the proper treatment. Marketing diseases and then
promoting drugs to treat those diseases is now common practice in the pharmaceutical world, made all the more lucrative with DTC advertising.

Children's problems constitute a growing market for psychotropic drugs. Ritalin
for attention-deficit/hyperactivity disorder (ADHD) has a long history (Conrad,
1975) but perhaps now can be seen as a pioneer drug for children's behavior prob-

lems. While the public may be ambivalent about using drugs for troubled children (McLeod et al., 2004), a wide array of psychotropic drugs are now prescribed for children, especially stimulants and antidepressants (Olfson et al., 2002; Thomas et al., 2006). Whatever the benefits or risks, this has become big business for the drug industry. According to a recent survey, spending on behavior drugs for children and adolescents rose 77 percent from 2000 through 2003. These drugs are now the fastest growing type of medication taken by children, eclipsing antibiotics and asthma treatments (Freudenheim, 2004).

At the other end of the life spectrum, it is likely that the $400 billion Medicare drug benefit, despite its limits, may increase pharmaceutical treatments for a range of elder problems as well. This policy shift in benefits is likely to encourage pharmaceutical companies to expand their markets by promoting more drug solutions for elders.

Genetics and Enhancement

We are at the dawn of the age of genomic medicine. While there has been a great investment in the Human Genome Project, and a celebration when the draft of the human genome was completed in 2000, most of genetic medicine remains on the level of potential rather than current practice. For example, we have known about the specific genes for cystic fibrosis and Huntington disease for a decade, but the knowledge has yet to translate into improvements in treatment. Thus far genetics has made its impact mostly in terms of the ability to test for gene mutations, carriers, or genetic anomalies. Despite the publicity given to genetic studies (Conrad, 1997), we have learned that only a few disorders and traits are linked to a single gene, and that genetic complexity (several genes operating together, gene-environment interactions) is the rule (Conrad, 1999). But I have little doubt that genomics will become increasingly important in the future and affect medicalization.

Although the impact of genetic medicine on medicalization still lies in the realm of potential, it is virtually certain that when the genetic contributors to problems such as obesity and baldness are identified, genetic tests and eventually treatments will follow. Obesity is an increasing problem in our society and has become more medicalized recently in a number of ways, from a spate of epidemiological studies showing the increase in obesity and body fat among Americans to the huge rise in intestinal bypass operations. Today physicians prescribe exercise and the Atkins or South Beach diet; it is possible that in the future there could be medical interventions in the genes (assuming they can be identified) that recognize satiation. Gene therapy has not yet succeeded for many problems, but one can imagine the rush to genetic doctors if there were a way to manipulate genes to control one's weight. We know that baldness often has a genetic basis, and with Rogaine and hair transplants it has already begun to be medicalized. However, with some kind of medical genetic intervention that either stops baldness or regenerates hair, one could see baldness move directly into the medical sphere, perhaps as a genetic "hair growth disorder."

A large area for growth in genetics and medicalization will be what I have termed "biomedical enhancement" (see chapter 4). Again, this is still in the realm of potential, but the potential is real. There is a great demand for enhancements, be they for our children, our bodies, or our mental and social abilities. Medical enhancements are a growing form of such interventions. One can imagine the potential of genetic enhancements in bodily characteristics such as height, musculature, shape, or color; in abilities such as memory, eyesight, hearing, and strength; or in talents (e.g., perfect pitch for music) and physical performance. Enhancements could become a huge market in a society in which individuals often seek an edge or a leg up. While many genetic improvements may remain in the realm of science fiction, there are sufficient monetary incentives for biotechnology companies to invest in pursuing genetic enhancements.

As discussed in chapter 4, the case of human growth hormone highlights the potentials and pitfalls of biomedical enhancement. The potential market for genetic enhancements is enormous. It has long been believed that shortness is devalued and engenders social problems for short individuals, although recent research has called this into question (e.g., Kelnar et al., 1999). Still, many parents are concerned that their children will be too short and go to a physician for hGH treatment. Since synthetic hGH became available in 1985, there has been a treatment available. Up until the last couple of years, Protropin, manufactured by Genentech, which is approved for only a limited number of specific growth disorders, has been used on an off-label basis to treat children with idiopathic short stature (i.e., shortness with an unknown cause). A relatively limited number of potentially short children were treated with Protropin, but the number is apt to grow because the FDA recently approved an Eli Lilly growth hormone, Humatrope, for use for short-statured children in the shortest 1.2 percent of the population. This is a potential market of 400,000 children. Ironically, as more children are treated and grow beyond the shortest 1.2 percent line, others will drop below this percentage threshold, thus creating an increasing pool of eligible children, beyond the 400,000 originally estimated. There are several lessons for biomedical enhancement here. First, a private market for enhancements for children, even involving significant expense, exists and can be tapped by biotechnology companies. Second, biotechnology companies, like pharmaceutical companies, will work to increase the size of their markets. Third, the promotion and use of biomedical enhancements will increase medicalization of human problems, in this case short stature. Imagine if genetic interventions to increase a child's height were available.

We do not yet have biotechnology companies promoting genetic enhancements, but we will. Biotech companies are already poised to use DTC advertising to promote genetic tests. They will employ many of the same marketing strategies as the pharmaceutical companies, which is no surprise, because many of them are one in the same or linked. The promotion of genetic tests may also contribute to medicalization. A positive finding on a genetic test—that one has a gene for a particular problem (cancer, alcoholism)—may create a new medicalized status, that of "potentially ill." This can have an impact on one's identity, social status, and insurability, and it may create new categories of precancer, prealcoholism, or similar labels. This could expand medical surveillance (D. Armstrong, 1995) and the medical gaze.

CONSUMERS

In our changing medical system, consumers of health care have become major players. As health care becomes more commodified and subject to market forces, medical care has become more like other products and services. We now are consumers, choosing health insurance plans, purchasing health care in the marketplace, and selecting institutions of care. Hospitals and health care institutions now compete for patients as consumers. I will briefly cite several examples of how consumers have become a major factor in medicalization: cosmetic surgery, adult ADHD, hGH therapy, and the rise in pharmaceutical advertisements.

Cosmetic surgery is the exemplar of consumerism in medicine (Sullivan, 2001). Procedures from tummy tucks to liposuction to nose jobs to breast augmentation have become big medical business. The body has become a project, from minor touch-up to "extreme makeover," and medicine has become the vehicle for improvement. In a sense the whole body has become medicalized, piece by piece. To use just an example that was discussed in chapter 6, the number of breast implants continuously increased until the silicone implant risk scare, when the market for implants plummeted. But with the introduction of apparently safer saline implants, breast augmentations increased by 90 percent from 1990 to 2000. According to the American Society for Aesthetic Plastic Surgery, in 2004 there were 334,052 breast augmentations in the United States (up 19% from the previous year), making this procedure the second most popular cosmetic surgery following liposuction. While plastic surgeons do promote breast augmentation as a product (current cost about $3,000), the medicalization of breasts and bodies is driven largely by the consumer market. Overall, 11.9 million Americans had cosmetic medical procedures in 2004, a 49 percent rise from the previous year and a more than 300 percent rise since 1997 (ASAPS, 2004). While the media and professional promotion fuel demand, virtually all of these procedures are paid for directly out of the consumer's pocket.

Since the early 1970s, Ritalin has been a common treatment for ADHD (formerly known as hyperactivity) in children. However, in the 1990s a new phenomenon emerged: adult ADHD. Researchers had shown for years that whatever ADHD was, it often persisted beyond childhood, but in the 1990s we began to see adults coming to physicians asking to be evaluated for ADHD and treated with medication. This was in part a result of several books, including one with the evocative title *Driven to Distraction* (Hallowell and Ratey, 1994), along with a spate of popular articles that publicized the disorder. Adults would come to physicians and say, "My son is ADHD and I was just like him," "I can't get my life organized, I must have ADHD," or "I know I'm ADHD, I read it in a book." Because Ritalin for adult attention problems is an off-label use of the medication, the pharmaceutical companies cannot directly advertise either the disorder or its treatment, but there are other ways to publicize the disorder. There are any number of Internet websites describing adult ADHD and its treatment, and the advocacy group Children and Adults with Attention-Deficit/Hyperactivity Disorder (CHADD) has become a strong advocate for identifying and treating adult ADHD. It is well known that CHADD gets much of its funding from the drug industry. Even so, CHADD is a consumer oriented group and, along with adults seeking ADHD treatment, has become a major force in what I have called "the medicalization of underperformance."

Adult ADHD is only one example of what Arthur Barsky and Jonathan Boros (1995) identified as the public's decreased tolerance for mild symptoms and benign problems. Individuals' self-medicalization is becoming increasingly common, with patients taking their troubles to physicians and often asking directly for a specific medical solution. A prominent example of this has been the increasing medicalization of unhappiness (Shaw and Woodward, 2004) and expansive treatment with antidepressants.

Nonprofit consumer groups like CHADD, the National Alliance for the Mentally Ill (NAMI), and the Human Growth Foundation have become strong supporters for medical treatments for the human problems for which they advocate. These consumer advocacy groups are comprised of families, patients, and others concerned with the particular disorder. However, these consumer groups are often supported financially by pharmaceutical companies. CHADD received support from Novartis, manufacturer of Ritalin; the Human Growth Foundation is at least in part funded by Genentech and Eli Lilly, makers of the hGH drugs; and between 1996 and 1999, NAMI received nearly $12 million from pharmaceutical companies (Silverstein, 1999). Spokespeople from such groups often take strong stances supporting pharmaceutical research and treatment, raising the question of where consumer advocacy begins and pharmaceutical promotion ends. This reflects the power of corporations in shaping and sometimes co-opting advocacy groups.

The Internet has become an important consumer vehicle. On the one hand, all pharmaceutical companies and most advocacy groups have websites replete with consumer-oriented information. These often include self-administered screening tests to help individuals decide whether they might have a particular disorder or benefit from some medical treatment. In addition, there are thousands of bulletin boards, chat rooms, and web pages where individuals can share information about illness, treatments, complaints, and services (Hardey, 2001). This has for many individuals transformed illness from a private experience to a more public one. On these websites people who have similar ailments can connect and share information in new ways, which, despite the pitfalls of misinformation, empower them as consumers of medical care. Both corporate and grassroots websites can generate an increased demand for services and disseminate medical perspectives far beyond professional or even national boundaries.

In our current medical age, consumers have become increasingly vocal and active in their desire and demand for services. Individuals as consumers rather than patients help shape the scope of, and sometimes the demand for, medical treatments for human problems.[1]

MANAGED CARE

Over the past two decades, managed-care organizations or their successors have come to dominate health care delivery in the United States, largely in response to rising health care costs. Managed care requires preapprovals for medical treatment and sets limits on some types of care. This has given third-party payers more leverage and has often constrained both the care given by doctors and the care received by patients. To a degree, managed care has commercialized medicine and encouraged medical care organizations and doctors to emphasize profits over patient care. But this matter is complex, for in some instances managed care constrains medical care and in other cases provides incentives for more profitable care.

In terms of medicalization, managed care is both an incentive and a constraint. This is clearly seen in the psychiatric realm. Managed care has severely reduced the amount of insurance coverage for psychotherapy available to individuals with mental and emotional problems (Shore and Beigel, 1996), but it has been much more liberal with paying for psychiatric medications. Thus, managed care has become a factor in the increasing uses of psychotropic medications among adults and children (Goode, 2002). It seems likely that physicians prescribe pharmaceutical treatments for psychiatric disorders knowing that these are the types of medical interventions covered under managed-care plans, thus accelerating psychotropic treatments for human problems.

In the 1980s I would frequently say to my students that one of the limits on the medicalization of obesity is that Blue Cross/Blue Shield (then a dominant insurance/managed-care company) would not pay for gastric bypass operations. This is no longer the case. Many managed-care organizations have concluded that it is a better financial investment to cover gastric bypass surgery for a "morbidly obese" person than to pay for the treatment of all the potential medical sequelae including diabetes, stroke, heart conditions, and musculoskeletal problems. The number of gastric bypass and similar surgeries in the United States has risen from 20,000 in 1965 to 103,000 in 2003, with over 140,000 estimated in 2004 (Grady, 2004). In the context of the so-called obesity epidemic (Abelson and Kennedy, 2004), bypass operations are becoming an increasingly common way to treat the problem of extreme overweight, with the threshold for treatment decreasing and becoming more inclusive. The recent Medicare policy shift declaring obesity a disease could further expand the number of medical claims for the procedure. As the New York Times reported, "The surgery has become big business and medical centers are scrambling to start programs" (Grady, 2004: D1).

But managed-care organizations affect medicalization by what they don't cover as well. When there is a demand for certain procedures and insurance coverage is not forthcoming, private markets for treatment emerge (Conrad and Leiter, 2004). As noted earlier, until recently hGH was approved for use only with the very few children who have a growth hormone deficiency. The FDA approval of Humatrope expanded the number of children eligible for growth hormone treatment to at least 400,000. It will be interesting to see whether managed-care organizations will cover the expensive hGH treatments for these children.

In effect, managed care is a selective double-edged sword for medicalization. Viagra and erectile dysfunction provide an interesting example. Some managed-care organizations' drug benefits cover (with co-pays) either four or six pills a month. While it is unclear how these insurance companies came up with these figures, it seems evident that managed-care strictures both bolster and constrain the medicalization of male sexual dysfunction. Increasingly, though, managed-care organizations are an arbiter of what is deemed medically appropriate or inappropriate treatment.

MEDICALIZATION IN THE NEW MILLENNIUM

The engines behind increasing medicalization are shifting from the medical profession, interprofessional or organizational contests, and social movements and interest groups to biotechnology, consumers, and managed-care organizations. Doctors are still gatekeepers for medical treatment, but their role has become more subordinate in the expansion or contraction of medicalization.[2] In short, the engines of medicalization have proliferated and are now driven more by commercial and market interests than by professional claims-makers.

The definitional center of medicalization remains constant, but the availability and promotion of new pharmaceutical and potential genetic treatments are increasingly drivers for new medical categories (cf. Horwitz, 2002). While it is still true that medicalization is not technologically determined, commercial and corporate stakeholders play a major role in how the technology will or won't be framed. For example, if a new pharmaceutical treatment comes to market, the drug industry may well pursue the promotion of new or underused medical definitions to legitimate the product (e.g., Paxil and SAD/GAD), attempt to change the definitions of a disorder (e.g., hGH and idiopathic short stature), or expand the definitions and lower the treatment threshold of an existing medicalized problem (e.g., Viagra and erectile dysfunction).[3]

Blood pressure became medicalized in the twentieth century. Elevated blood pressure was first medicalized on the conceptual level as hypertension, then on the organizational level through blood pressure screenings, and finally by physicians in their diagnosis of hypertension as a risk factor for illness and prescribing pharmaceutical treatment (Kawachi and Conrad, 1996). Of particular interest here are the questions surrounding what constitutes hypertension (e.g., at what point measured blood pressure is defined as diseased) and the role of drug treatment in the changing thresholds of potential pathology. What has been termed "mild hypertension" is a debatable area, but it has largely not been treated with antihypertensive medications. However, the American Society of Hypertension has recently engaged in a campaign, financed by the pharmaceutical companies, to redefine hypertension in terms of a broader syndrome. Hypertension, which is a risk factor for cardiovascular disease, is commonly treated with pharmaceuticals and constitutes a $17 billion annual market (Saul, 2006). By the current definition, which encompasses about 65 million Americans, a blood pressure reading of 140/90 or above constitutes hypertension. But the pharmaceutical companies have been promoting a new designation of "prehypertensive," defined as blood pressure readings of 120/80. This expanded definition, combined with other cardiovascular risk factors, would increase the potential hypertensive drug market by about 30 million people. The pharmaceutical companies' obvious self-interest in this matter was the subject of a recent editorial in the New York Times (2006). Such an expansion of hypertension is a controversial notion among cardiologists and other physicians (Saul, 2006), but clearly it would enlarge the market for antihypertensive medications and thus expand the swath of the medicalization of blood pressure.

A recent, little-known example illustrates the promotion of new disorders. Avanir, a pharmaceutical company, is attempting to get FDA approval for its drug Neurodex for a disorder the company is calling "pseudobulbar affect," or PBA. According to Avanir, "Pseudobulbar affect is a condition characterized by episodes of uncontrollable laughing and/or crying that may be inappropriate or unrelated to the situation at hand" (www.pseudobulbar.com), which can be caused by a variety of neurological diseases or injuries (e.g., multiple sclerosis, amyotropic lateral sclerosis, stroke). One doctor described it as "pathologic laughter that is devoid of any inner sense of joy and pathologic weeping [devoid] of any feeling of inner sorrow" (Pollack, 2005). The drug company has completed two clinical trials demonstrating that Neurodex reduces unwanted laughter and crying, although it also has some unpleasant side effects. Critics question whether this is a syndrome warranting drug treatment; some have suggested that the laughing and crying is a relatively minor problem for those with life-threatening diseases. Avanir has hired neurologists and psychiatrists to promote pseudobulbar affect as a treatable illness, sponsored a quarterly newsletter "PBA Update," set up a website, and considered starting a patient advocacy group (Pollack, 2005). The company's CEO, Dr. Gerald J. Yakatan, is surprisingly direct when discussing the promotion of the disorder and its treatment. He compares PBA with erectile dysfunction and ADHD: "Before there were drugs, these conditions didn't exist" (quoted in Pollack, 2005). Avanir estimates on its website that more than a million Americans may have pseudobulbar affect. My point here is not to debate whether PBA is a real illness but rather to illustrate how a pharmaceutical company may promote an illness in order to sell the treatment for it. This is a clear example of medicalization in process; one key to the outcome will be whether or not the FDA approves the drug for treatment of PBA.

Drug companies are having an increasing impact on the boundaries of the normal and the pathological, becoming active agents of social control. This is worrisome for a number of reasons, but perhaps especially "because corporations are ultimately more responsible to their shareholders than to patients; shareholder desires are often at odds with patients' needs for rational drug prescribing" (Wilkes et al., 2000). It may well be to the shareholders' advantage for pharmaceutical companies to promote medications for an ever-increasing array of human problems, but this in no way ensures that these constitute improvements in health and medical care. And what is the impact of the new engines of medicalization on the rising costs of health care?

In a culture of increasingly market-driven medicine, consumers, biotechnological corporations, and medical services interact in complex ways that affect social norms in changing definitions of behaviors and interventions. The relationship between normative changes and medicalization runs in both directions. For example, changing norms about breast augmentation are one cause of medicalization, while at the same time the processes of medicalization themselves lead to changes in the social norms surrounding breast enhancements. Similarly, advertisements for Viagra have destigmatized male erectile dysfunction, while a normalized notion of erectile dysfunction has increased the consumer demand for Viagra.

I would be remiss if I did not note here the gendered nature of much corporatized medicalization. This should be no surprise, because women's bodies have long been objects of medical control (Riska, 2003). We are now seeing the expansion of largely gendered markets for medicalization, such as Viagra and Ritalin for males and Prozac and cosmetic surgery for females (e.g., Blum and Stracuzzi, 2004). And there may be more coming, with growing markets for andropause and baldness targeting men and the pharmaceutical industry's ardent search for a female equivalent of Viagra. While corporate medicalizers might wish to include both men and women to increase their market potential, gender segmentation is a propitious strategy for defining problems and promoting medical solutions, both exploiting and reinforcing gender boundaries.

Medicalization is prevalent in the United States, but it is increasingly an international phenomenon. This is partly the result of the expanding hegemony of Western biomedicine, but it is facilitated by multinational drug companies and the global reach of mass media and the Internet. As John McKinlay and Lisa Marceau note, "Transnational corporations involved in the globalization of medicine (pharmaceuticals, services, medical insurance, and biotechnology) generate local demand for services" (2002: 399). The pharmaceutical companies' introduction and promotion of "mild depression" as an illness in Japan has resulted in a dramatic rise in SSRI treatment since 1999 (Schulz, 2004). Furthermore, cyberspace knows no national boundaries, expediting the dissemination of medical knowledge, commercial promotion, and consumer desires. Perspectives that germinate in Boston today are available in Cairo or Moscow by the evening and in Calcutta and Yogyakarta, Indonesia, the next day. We have no idea yet what the Internet's impact is on the local and global nature of medical categories and treatments, but it is a safe assumption that medicalization will increase with globalization.

Professional and public concern about medicalization may be growing as well. The *British Medical Journal* devoted nearly an entire issue (2002) to medicalization topics, and we increasingly see the term "medicalization" used in the popular press. A outstanding example of this is the *Seattle Times'* five-part investigative series, "Suddenly Sick: The Hidden Big Business behind Your Doctor's Diagnosis" (Kelleher and Wilson, 2005). For years, when I talked with people about medicalization, I would always need to explain in detail what I meant. Now most people quickly understand what the term means. But despite the increased awareness and openness to the issue, we also need to develop our own understandings of medicalization in new and deeper ways.

Social scientists and critics need to turn their attention in medicalization research to the emergent engines of medicalization. This means examining the impact of biotechnological discoveries, the influence of pharmaceutical industry marketing and promotion, the role of consumer demand, the facilitating and constraining aspects of managed care and health insurance, the impact of the Internet, the changing role of the medical profession and physicians, and the pockets of medical and popular resistance to medicalization. This means supplementing the social constructionist studies with political economic perspectives. Medicalization still doesn't occur without social actors doing something to make an entity medical, but the engines that are driving medicalization have changed, and we need to refocus our sociological eye as the medicalization train moves into the twenty-first century.

CHAPTER EIGHT

Medicalization and Its Discontents

I have argued throughout this book that the medicalization of society has increased and that powerful social forces within and outside of medicine are fueling this expansion. There will undoubtedly be some who will herald the expansion of medicine as a sign of social progress and a wholesale benefit to humankind. There is no doubt that medicine and even some forms of medicalization have made significant contributions to the welfare of human beings. But my concern in this book is with the widespread medicalization, perhaps overmedicalization, of human conditions, a trend that shows no signs of abatement. In this chapter I discuss medicalization's social consequences, the controversies that surround it, and some pockets of resistance. I also outline my concerns about the continuing trend toward medicalizing human problems.

Before I discuss the social consequences of medicalization, I want to reiterate two important points. First, I do not argue in this book whether or not a given problem is "really" medical. Primarily, I don't know what "really" means in this context, and additionally, I do not have the ability or desire to adjudicate whether some malady is truly medical, by whatever standards it might be evaluated. Thus, my claim is simply that these problems are not *inherently* medical but have become medicalized, and this medicalization has important social consequences. Second, I do not deny that there may be some extreme cases of problems that have a biological or physiological basis, but that does not necessarily mean that all cases of that problem have a biological basis. Having a biological basis does not make something ipso facto a medical problem; left-handedness or the growth of some people to 7 feet tall or more may have a genetic basis, and the onset of puberty may have a hormonal source, but these conditions are not defined as medical problems. In other cases, perhaps some small subset of those diagnosed with a given condition have a physiological anomaly that becomes a justification for widespread treatment for a particular malady. As one example, it is certainly possible that a small proportion of children with a diagnosis of attention deficit hyperactivity disorder may have a discernable neurological problem, but the identification and diagnosis of ADHD goes far beyond these few children and includes a huge number of children with no identifiable neurological disorder. This kind of "medicalization spread" occurs for many other problems as well. The social consequences inhere in the medicalized category and diagnosis and are not dependent on the existence or absence of biophysiological evidence.

SOCIAL CONSEQUENCES

It is conceivable that a reader could get this far in the book and ask the question, So what? There has been widespread medicalization, but what does it matter? Which social issues surround medicalization, and why should this trend be an object of concern?

What I discuss here are issues that inhere in the medicalization of human problems independent of any potential "benefits" from medicalization. Put another way, there are certain social consequences of medicalization irrespective of any attendant medical or social benefit.

More than a quarter of a century ago, when I first wrote about the medicalization of deviance (Conrad, 1975; Conrad and Schneider, 1980: 246–52), I conceptualized the brighter and darker sides of medicalization. The broader focus here on the medicalization of society requires us to rethink some of these consequences.

Before I outline some of the social ramifications that make me skeptical of the medicalization of society, I need to present a few caveats. There no doubt are some benefits to medicalization. On the social side, medicalization allows for extension of the sick role to a wider range of maladies and thus can reduce individual blame for the problem (e.g., in cases of ADHD, alcoholism, and erectile dysfunction). Some forms of medicalization (e.g., Alcoholics Anonymous, interventions for anorexia) may reduce stigma or allow individuals to function better in society. In some controversial areas, medicalization may be a form of harm reduction (Shell-Duncan, 2001). On the medical side, many of us know individuals whose life has been significantly improved by psychoactive medications, who are no longer depressed, disoriented, or disordered thanks to medical interventions. Some individuals undoubtedly have been helped by medical treatments for obesity, anorexia, menopause, ADHD, and erectile dysfunction. And one might even argue that, in some cases, biomedical enhancements with interventions such as human growth hormone or breast implants have improved the self-esteem or life opportunities of individuals. These particular benefits should not be dismissed, but they also do not necessarily justify the social consequences of widespread medicalization. In chapters 2 through 5 I have already pointed to some specific ramifications of medicalization for particular life issues or problems; here I identify several additional troubling consequences of medicalization in a broader social context.

The Pathologization of Everything

One of my main concerns with the widespread medicalization of society is its transformation of many human differences into pathologies. Differences in learning styles become learning disabilities or ADHD; divergences in sexual desires or performance become sexual dysfunctions; extremes of behavior become sexual, shopping, or Internet addictions (e.g., Quinn, 2001); and individual differences become diagnoses such as social phobia or idiopathic short stature. We have long turned normal life events into medical events, from conception to childbirth to menopause to aging. We are now turning breast size, shortness, and male baldness into problems that are subject to medical enhancements. In the not-so-distant future we will likely attempt to use genetic interventions to design babies who are free from characteristics we deem pathological, such as short height, proneness to "addictions," low academic intelligence, or athletic clumsiness. Virtually any human difference is susceptible to being considered a form of pathology, a diagnosable disorder, and subject to medical intervention. As Nancy Press notes, "Medicalization pathologizes what might otherwise be considered as simply variations in normal human functioning" (2006: 138). The great danger here is that transforming all difference into pathology diminishes our tolerance for and appreciation of the diversity of human life.

More than a decade ago a physician named Clifton Meador published an article called "The Last Well Person" in the *New England Journal of Medicine*. In a fictional scenario set in the not-too-distant future, Meador depicted a 53-year-old professor of first-year algebra at a small college in the Midwest. No matter how much medical evaluation he received, doctors were unable to find anything wrong with him. He was the last person in the world for whom this was true. Meador warned that if the behavior of doctors and the public continues unabated, "eventually every well person would be labeled sick" (1994: 441). This is even more true today (cf. Hadler, 2004).

In a culture in which health has become a high-value asset, it should not be surprising that life problems have become medical pathologies. One of the ironies of our culture is that no matter how much health is improved (as evidenced by decreased mortality rates, increased life expectancy, and improved health care), the reporting of health problems continues to rise (Bury, 2005). In part this is due to the expansion of available diagnoses; as noted in the opening of the book, now-common maladies such as ADHD, anorexia, chronic fatigue syndrome, post-traumatic stress disorder, panic disorder, fetal alcohol syndrome, premenstrual syndrome, and sudden infant death syndrome were not even heard of forty years ago. And as some commentators remind us, Americans have also become less tolerant of minor physical symptoms and uncomfortable body states and thus have become important advocates for medicalization (Barsky and Boros, 1995). One can only wonder if hypochondria is still a viable classification, given the huge increase in available medical diagnoses for individual troubles (Segal, 2005).

In the early twenty-first century, physicians are not necessarily the most active promoters of pathologization, although they are certainly important gatekeepers to diagnoses and medical treatment. The pharmaceutical industry has promoted new definitions of pathology while consumers have frequently sought diagnoses and medical treatments. Medicalization is not, nor ever has been, "medical imperialism" but is rather an increasingly complex interplay of various social actors.

Medical Definitions of Normality

Medical designations are increasingly defining what is "normal," expected, and acceptable in life. Sharon Kaufman and her colleagues have shown how changes in the availability and thresholds of medical interventions have transformed our view of normal aging and what constitutes routine clinical care: "It is through an ethics of normalcy that expectations about long lives and expectations about routine medical treatment come together. It is unacceptable to die at 71, or 81, or 91 if one can utilize routine medical care to stave off death and restore health" (2004: 736). But it is not only with aging that medicine has changed what is now deemed normal. Several examples presented in the book suggest the role of medical norms in setting social norms.

For instance, impotence and sexual performance difficulties have in all likelihood been human afflictions for eons. But with the introduction of Viagra and its fellow medications for erectile dysfunction (ED), the expectations of sexual performance have grown, especially among older men. Men now can expect to be sexually active until well into old age, not always to the joy of their partners (see Loe,

2004). The medicalization of ED has changed expectations about male sexual performance. As physician Steven B. Levine, an expert in sexuality, points out, "We used to treat older people as though sex was not possible; and now we've flipped-flopped and transmitted the message that everyone is supposed to have fantastic sex forever. Over age 50, the quality of sex depends much more on the overall quality of the relationship than it does for young couples" (quoted in Hoberman, 2005: 145).

There have always been people who were shy in social situations or who have had difficulty speaking in public settings (S. Scott, 2006). In the past this social reticence was typically considered characterological for these individuals and part of the normal range of human personality. But the pharmaceutical company Glaxo-SmithKline has promoted "social anxiety disorder" (SAD), previously considered a rare psychiatric condition, as a common ailment, with its drug Paxil as its treatment. At one point SAD was claimed to affect one in eight Americans. The drug company began a campaign to raise public awareness of SAD and "to reshape public perceptions about shyness and uneasiness in social situations" (Moynihan and Cassels, 2005: 120). Such social uneasiness was now out of the range of normal human behavior and had become a medical entity in need of treatment (cf. S. Scott, 2006).

Humatrope, a form of human growth hormone (hGH), has been approved for treating children without a diagnosed growth hormone deficiency but who are in the 1.2 lowest percentile of potential height. We can anticipate that, given this "remedy," the expectations for normal height may change. People are now viewed as being "too short" rather than normal within a range of heights. Whatever treatment threshold is set for hGH treatment is arbitrary; it is not inconceivable that the threshold treatment will change and at some point perhaps the shortest 3.5 percent or 10 percent of individuals will be labeled abnormal and thus subject to potential medical intervention. What is significant here is not that hundreds of thousands of short children will be treated with hGH (which is unlikely, given that the treatments are very expensive and currently not covered by health insurance) but the fact that medicine has defined the norm of what is "too short." Ironically, hGH may make some children a few inches taller, which will allow other children to fall into the designated low percentile range—thus continually expanding the pool of potentially treatable children.

Of concern with these three examples, and in a different way with menopause and hypertension, is that pharmaceutical companies are defining, either directly by setting numbers or indirectly by promoting diagnoses, what is deemed normal or abnormal. What is worrying, of course, is that the pharmaceutical companies have an investment in creating these new norms in order to market their products. Using powerful resources like direct-to-consumer advertising, the pharmaceutical industry has increased its influence in defining what is normal, expected, and even acceptable in society (Conrad and Leiter, 2005).

The Expansion of Medical Social Control

Social control is necessary for society to function; sociologists have long pointed out the importance of social regulation (Durkheim, 1933; Janowitz, 1975). In his classic formulation, Talcott Parsons (1951) pointed out the social control functions of medicine, especially in terms of managing and reintegrating people who are sick into society.

But as Irving K. Zola (1972) and others (Conrad, 1979) have shown, as medical jurisdiction has expanded, the reach of medical social control has widened. In one sense, the definition of medical norms is in itself a cultural form of social control, in that it creates new expectations for bodies, behavior, and health. This control is manifested in how medical expectations set the boundaries for behavior and well-being as well has how medical norms guide behavior. One need only think of how a diagnosis like fetal alcohol syndrome (E. Armstrong, 2003) has changed the behavior of pregnant women or people's views of pregnant women who drink even a single glass of wine.

Medical surveillance (D. Armstrong, 1995), another expanded form of medical social control, has led an increasing number of individuals to become objects of medical interest, even though they may not be currently ill. Often these individuals are deemed at risk for a disease and monitored to ascertain any changes in their risk. This is typically the case with blood pressure, cholesterol, or prostate-specific antigen or PSA levels, as these are known as risk factors for strokes, heart disease, or prostate cancer (see also Klawiter, 1998, on risk and breast cancer surveillance). By no means do I imply that such monitoring is not beneficial to individuals; I only point out that these are examples of the increased role surveillance medicine plays in the social control of behavior. In addition to focusing on those that are ill, the medical vision now includes an increasingly large number of people who are regarded as potentially ill. (More will be said about that later.) When genes for susceptibility to a particular disease are identified, this information will likely be used to swell the population of the potentially ill, and individuals will be monitored for the potential manifestation of the disease or disorder (Conrad, 2000).

Finally, medical social control includes various forms of medical therapies, especially pharmaceuticals and surgical interventions, that change the behavior, body, or psychic state of individuals. Pharmaceuticals have long been considered a form of medical social control of deviance, and their use is expanding to modify everyday behavior, mood, sexuality, learning abilities, and so forth. Medications like Prozac, Viagra, and hGH only extend what has long been medicine's province. Surgery can be another form of medical social control. The increasing use of gastric bypass operations for obesity, the rising number of breast implants (Conrad and Jacobson, 2003), and other forms of cosmetic surgery (Sullivan, 2001) are medical interventions that reshape bodies to make them more socially acceptable. Medicalization is key to these types of social control; without the problem being medicalized, physicians could not legitimately perform these kinds of procedures.

One social implication of increased medical social control is that more forms of behavior are no longer deemed the responsibility of the individual. That is, when the cause is seen as biological and subject to "medical excuse," the individual is no longer considered responsible for the behavior. The social response moves from being punitive to being therapeutic. The scope of medical excuses is wide: it ranges from medical diagnosis and treatment for problems in elementary school all the way to the insanity defense for capital crimes. While in many cases (as with alcoholism or drug addiction) this may be a more humane approach, it also extends the range of behaviors for which people are no longer considered responsible. This dislocation of responsibility has certain social ramifications (see Conrad and Schneider, 1992).

A Narrow Focus on Individuals Rather Than Social Context

It has long been observed that the clinical gaze or the clinical medical model focuses on the individual rather than the social context. After all, the individual for the most part is the target of medical (though not public health) interventions. What I have previously called "the individualization of social problems" remains a consequence of medicalization. This isn't news to observers of medicalization, so I will treat it only briefly here.

The general mode is to solve the problem in the individual, not the society: treat the individual with alcoholism or the disruptive child with ADHD rather than intervene in the environment that produces alcohol abuse or the school system that deems the child troublesome or troubled. (For a contextualized view, see Hart et al., 2006.) Medicalization can obscure the social forces that influence well-being. For example, by focusing completely on the neurobiological features of depression, this condition is viewed increasingly as being genetic, and it is treated predominantly with antidepressants, while the social environments that frequently feed depression are not altered (Horwitz, 2002). In a different way this is true with Viagra and ED, with a fix in physiology rather than in relationships. The focus on the individual has reinforced the proclivity of treating complex societal problems with technological fixes (e.g., a medical, surgical, or pharmaceutical intervention) rather than by changing the social structure.

Disability provides a good example. The medicalized view of disability focuses on the individual's physical impairments rather than on the disabling features of society (see Oliver, 1996). For decades the goal of intervention was "rehabilitation." However useful this medicalized approach may have been in improving individual function, with the rise of the disability movement the focus of intervention shifted to removing barriers in the disabling social environment, in the form of accommodations like curb cuts in sidewalks, Braille and floor bells in elevators, and ramps in public buildings. A particularly interesting example has been the deaf community's campaign against cochlear implants in children as the unnecessary medicalization of deafness. Many advocates see deafness as a culture, not a disease, and so deem medical interventions in children to be inappropriate (Crouch, 1997).

While the clinical medical model focuses on the individual, the cutting-edge fields of scientific medicine, neuroscience and genetics, reflect and reinforce this view. Neuroscience, with research on the brain and brain functioning, will likely bring new treatments for new diseases, but the danger is that it will also become a justification for new areas of medicalization (Rose, 2005). Genetics, which has expanded enormously in the wake of the Human Genome Project, focuses on the level of DNA while typically ignoring the social environment necessary for genes to be expressed. Too often, genes are seen as *the* cause for a disorder; this creates the mirage that this bit of DNA is the primary cause of a problem (Conrad, 1999). A few studies have shown that the interaction between genetics and the environment is a more likely explanation for most human characteristics and ailments (Caspi et al., 2003). But medicalization reinforces the individualized approaches to social problems that are common in our society.

Consumers and Medical Markets

One of the most significant changes in medicalization in the past thirty years has been the emergence of consumers and medical markets. These are of course related, but they are not always connected.

Medical entrepreneurs, including pharmaceutical and biotechnology companies, along with some medical experts, have been marketing medical solutions for a range of human problems. In earlier chapters I presented Viagra, Paxil, hGH, and hormone replacement therapy as examples of pharmaceutical promotion that increases medicalization. In the United States (and New Zealand), DTC advertising is a major vehicle for promoting both diagnoses and the medications to treat them

(Conrad and Leiter, 2005). The common tagline, "Ask your doctor if [Viagra, Paxil, Zoloft, etc.] is right for you," reflects the new relation among pharmaceutical manufacturers, consumers, and physicians. Many of these companies hire experts to promote a disorder and so expand the market for their product (Moynihan and Cassels, 2005). Pharmaceutical companies promote their products on websites that include simple questionnaires to allow consumers to determine whether they have a disorder and should consult a physician to treat it. While pharmaceutical companies have long been involved in medicalization, their role is now much greater and more direct. For example, while pharmaceutical companies in the 1970s advertised drugs for hyperactive, restless, and disruptive children, they were limited to advertising prescription medications only to physicians; now they can advertise directly to consumers and attempt to directly expand their markets.

When third parties (e.g., health insurance companies) pay for a promoted medication or medical procedure, we have what we call a "mediated" market (Conrad and Leiter, 2004): the market for the treatment is mediated by the coverage policy of the insurance company, government program, or managed-care organization. Thus, while advertising is direct medicalization, the market for the treatment is mediated by whether or not it is covered by insurance. Sometimes expansions or contractions in coverage can affect the amount of medicalization that occurs. It will be interesting to see, for example, what impact the new Medicare drug benefit will have on the medicalization of problems among older adults covered by the program.

Some medically promoted treatments and procedures are not covered by insurance; these direct markets are similar to markets for other goods and services in society (Conrad and Leiter, 2004). Several cases in this book (e.g., baldness treatments and breast augmentation) fit into this category. This growing commercialization—perhaps most especially in areas like cosmetic surgery and infertility treatments, but including interventions for conditions like idiopathic short stature—exemplifies a new market mentality in parts of medicine. Doctors have services to offer, and patients qua consumers are able to purchase them if they desire. One can find advertisements in magazines and on the Internet for such medical services; I recall reading several ads for breast enhancements (for less than $3,000!) in magazines like Cosmopolitan and noting on numerous websites that medical practices have connections directly with banks to arrange loans for cosmetic surgery. What we have is a fusion of increased medicalization and commercialized medicine. Medical services or treatments become commodities, much like any other product. This can be conceptualized as the business of medicalization.

But not all directly advertised medical services succeed. In 2000, many companies offered CT scans to the public with the promise of early detection of diseases like cancer or heart disease, with no doctor referral necessary. At first the demand was great; hundreds of body scanning clinics opened, large sums were spent on DTC advertising, and most centers had long waiting lists. By the end of 2004 the bubble had burst, and most centers had closed for lack of business. What happened? Professional societies warned that the scans would be problematic to interpret, would reveal innocuous findings, and would simply lead to more tests. With insurers refusing to cover the procedure, consumers were ultimately unwilling to pay $1,000 or more for a scan. The radiologists who had thought there was a huge market of people willing to pay were mistaken (Kolata, 2005). There appear to be limits to what consumers are willing to pay out of their own pockets for knowledge about their health. It will be interesting to see how consumers respond to the DNA tests that are now becoming available (Geller, 2006). Consumer demand for medical information may not, however, necessarily translate into specific medical disorders or treatments.

Consumers are playing an increasing role in medicalization in several ways. First, as mentioned, consumers encouraged by DTC advertising ask their doctor whether they have the disorder they saw in a magazine or on television, and perhaps they request a particular medication (Conrad and Leiter, 2005). Second, consumers can obtain medical products and services in both mediated and private markets. Third, consumers are coming to physicians and requesting treatment for self-diagnosed disorders. In chapter 3 we saw this trend exemplified with adult ADHD. Consumers also go to physicians with symptoms of "contested illnesses" like fibromyalgia (Barker, 2005b), chronic fatigue syndrome (L. Cooper, 1997), and multiple chemical sensitivity disorder (Kroll-Smith and Floyd, 1997). The legitimation these patients *qua* consumers are seeking is medicalization. The Internet has become a powerful vehicle for promoting medicalized definitions of a whole range of disorders (e.g., Salant and Santry, 2006). Virtually all disorders, contested or settled, have consumer websites, and many, though not all, promote increased medicalization of various life difficulties (Barker, 2005a).

In short, the marketing of medical solutions to life problems by medical entrepreneurs and the seeking and purchasing of these solutions by consumers have created an expanded industry in medicalization.

THE CHANGING ROLES OF PHYSICIANS

In the early writings on medicalization, physicians were depicted as central to the medicalization process. In terms of medical imperialism (Illich, 1976), professional dominance (Freidson, 1970), and medical claims-making (Conrad and Schneider, 1992), physicians were the major figures in medicalization. This is changing.

To be sure, the medical profession and physicians are still key players. The medical profession is often essential to the legitimation of new medical categories, as when professional bodies provide guidelines on new maladies; diagnoses become inscribed in official compendiums such as the DSM-IV; or some subgroup of physicians promotes a new disorder or a new treatment for a medical problem. But the primary engines of medicalization now also include consumers, insurers, and the biotechnological industry. Physicians haven't entirely been nudged aside, but they have been joined by other equally or more powerful players in the medicalization process (cf. Davis, 2006).

Physicians, however, do remain central as gatekeepers. For virtually all medicalized entities, it is physicians who administer the medical treatments. Thus, to get a diagnosis, obtain a prescription for medication, or have surgery, physicians are necessary. Others may encourage or constrain medical treatment, but physicians still retain crucial prerogatives in medical decision making. While the medical profession may be divided about whether chronic fatigue syndrome or fibromyalgia are treatable medical conditions, if a small number of physicians are willing to treat the disorder, it can become medicalized.

Physicians also retain the role of medical expert. While consumers and pharmaceutical companies may promote medicalization, physicians, as researchers and clinicians, are still deemed the authorities with regard to medical knowledge. Medical expertise still has significant cultural and legal cachet and is sought both by marketers and by consumers to support their positions on medicalized entities. This is why pharmaceutical companies seek medicoscientific justification to promote their products (Moynihan and Cassels, 2005) and those with contested illnesses seek medical allies to aid in their quest for illness legitimization (Kroll-Smith et al., 2000). Physicians remain the experts about medical knowledge and are necessary elements to medicalization. Neither companies nor individuals share their status in debates about diagnosis, illness, and treatment.

Although physicians are no longer the major promoters of medicalization, there is an area in which physicians often still push the boundaries of medicalization. One of the major goals of the medical profession, and of many physicians in practice, is to reduce the suffering of individuals. Indeed, this is one of the hallmarks of medicine and medical care. Yet one can also ask the question, What are the limits to medicine's role in reducing suffering? Clearly, medicine is not directly involved in reducing financial or ethnic suffering, but the limits of medical suffering are not clear. For example, I have heard physicians say they should treat school problems, shortness, small breasts, or disorganized adult lives with medical interventions because it reduces individuals' suffering. But where does the medical mandate to reduce suffering end? Will that mandate include anything related to the human body or mind that can be altered (Zola, 1972)? If a drug or a genetic or surgical intervention is introduced that can modify some problem whereby humans are suffering, will the attendant form of misery acquire a medical definition in order to use the intervention to reduce suffering? Will the treatment ultimately lead to the development of a diagnosis to justify the treatment? Are there any forms of individual suffering that affect the body, mind, or behavior that are beyond potential inclusion in the medical realm?

POCKETS OF RESISTANCE TO MEDICALIZATION

While the trends toward medicalization are clear, some pockets of resistance have appeared. The form and impact of each have been different.

The gay rights (now gay, lesbian, bisexual, transgender, and queer, or GLBTQ) movement is a classic example of resistance that has successfully changed the definition of homosexuality from an illness to a lifestyle to an orientation (Conrad and Schneider, 1992: 172–213). As discussed in chapter 5, despite some important cultural and scientific changes, the demedicalization of homosexuality continues to be sustained more than three decades after the 1974 American Psychiatric Association decision. In a vote of the membership, the APA decided to remove homosexuality as an illness from the DSM-III and replace it with a designation that included only individuals who were unhappy with their homosexual orientation.

Another successful challenge to medicalization has been the disability rights movement (Shapiro, 1994; Batavia and Schriner, 2001). As an extension of the Civil Rights movement, a new social movement was organized by and for people with disabilities in order to promote disability rights. While much of the emphasis of the movement was public access and combating discrimination in education and employment (culminating with the 1990 Americans with Disability Act, or ADA), one goal was also to transform disability from primarily a medical problem into a societal problem (cf. Oliver, 1996). Groups like the Independent Living Movement focused on what was necessary for people to function in society with and despite disability. The passage of the ADA and the continued persistence of members of the disability community have significantly altered the previous view that disability is fundamentally a medical problem. While recognizing the nature of physical and mental impairments, the disability rights movement still actively resists the medicalized concepts and control of disability.

Childbirth probably reached its zenith as a medicalized experience in the 1950s. Typically, at least in middle-class families, doctors delivered babies while the mother was sedated or under anesthesia, often in stirrups. Episiotomies and pain medications were routine, formula feeding was recommended for newborns, and so forth. In response to this situation, the "natural childbirth movement" arose, essentially developing and promoting ways to make birth less medicalized (Wertz and Wertz, 1989). The movement had considerable success, especially in promoting less intervention in childbirth, giving mothers more control and choices, and including fathers as labor coaches in the birth process. Hospitals began to offer more comfortable, even homelike, birthing rooms, and obstetricians gave women with uncomplicated births more choices in birthing strategies. Some women selected midwives for their births, and a few even chose to give birth at home. As important as these changes were, they affected middle- and upper-class women much more than poorer women. Significant to our analysis, these changes reflected reforms in medical childbirth rather than a demedicalization of childbirth. In the current era, we have a bifurcation of childbirth practices: some births are less medicalized (e.g., with childbirth classes, birthing rooms, and no anesthesia), while others are more medicalized (e.g., with internal fetal monitors, Cesarean sections, and attendant neonatal infant care units). In 2004 the C-section rate in the United States reached an all-time high of 29 percent (R. Rubin, 2005). Of interest, the number of *elective* C-sections has risen in recent years; this number now constitutes approximately 2.5 percent of all births, including a significant increase in first-time mothers (Health-Grades, 2005). In short, there has been resistance to medicalized childbirth, but the overall medicalization of childbirth is still predominant and may be increasing in some quarters.[1]

There have long been pockets of resistance to medicalized disorders like ADHD, including parents' groups and some activist organizations. In recent years the Church of Scientology has crusaded against the use of Ritalin (methylphenidate) and other stimulants for ADHD, with minimal success. Based on her interviews with mothers of children diagnosed with ADHD, Claudia Malacrida (2003) reports that in the United Kingdom there is some resistance from schools to treating children with stimulants, while in the United States, whatever resistance there exists comes from parents—not schools. Internet sites like the Alliance for Human Research Protection (www.ahrp.org) present critical viewpoints on the risks and widespread use of psychiatric medications, including stimulants, for children. A recent study suggests, however, that the prescribing of psychotropic medications for children's problems seems to have increased rapidly in the past decade (see chapter 6).

While obesity has been declared a health epidemic and gastric bypass operations are on the rise, organizations like National Association to Advance Fat Acceptance present an alternative to the medical definitions of overweight. These activists have mounted a protest movement against medical approaches to obesity, staunchly claiming that obesity is not a disease. They argue that bodies come in many sizes, and that health can be had at every size. (Crary, 2004). It is unclear whether this movement will have a significant impact on the definitions or treatment of obesity.

The advent of the Internet has created new areas for resistance to as well promotion of medicalization. One of the most interesting of these has been the emergence of pro-anorexia (pro-ana) websites. These are typically bulletin boards, chat rooms, or other interactive websites where people with anorexia and other eating disorders can communicate with one another. Unlike other illness-oriented websites, the pro-ana sites take a strong stance promoting anorexia as a lifestyle choice. They create a counternarrative to the medicalized view of anorexia (such as, "ana is my friend") and offer a distinct antirecovery stance toward the disorder (N. Fox et al., 2005). Many of the communications on these websites suggest that anorexia is a risky but fulfilling way of life; these sites include strategies on eating, purging, and how to be a better anorexic. They are careful to avoid the appearance of recruiting others into an anorexic way of life (warning messages abound that these sites are only for anorexics), but the rhetoric is definitely resistant to medicalized categories of eating disorders.

The pharmaceutical industry invests in medicalized categories when it wants to market a product to treat a particular disorder. The success of Viagra for erectile dysfunction has encouraged the pharmaceutical industry to find treatments for "female sexual dysfunction," or FSD (Hartley, 2003; Loe, 2004). A variety of companies have both promoted FSD as a disorder and conducted clinical trials for its treatment (Hartley, 2003). Psychologist Leonore Tiefer and some colleagues have critiqued the pharmaceutical approach to female sexuality and have organized research conferences and a group to counteract the medicalized view of female sexual problems (Tiefer, 2001a, 2001b). These advocates, who have formed the Working Group on a New View of Women's Sexual Problems, offer an alternative view to what they see as the reductionist medicalized framework (Tiefer, 2001b). As part of their campaign, they created an FSD Alert website (www.FSD-Alert.org). Here we have an alliance of feminists and professionals challenging the medicalization of female sexual difficulties, standing opposed to FSD promoters such as medical sexuality expert Irwin Goldstein and some pharmaceutical companies (Moynihan and Cassels, 2005).

As noted in chapter 6, risk scares such as with hormone replacement therapy or silicone breast implants can engender resistance to medicalization or at least to medicalized interventions. The potential adverse effects of medications, such as high blood pressure or odd structural abnormalities of hands and feet, may limit the use of human growth hormone as an antiaging medication (Weintraub, 2006). The recent reports of increased risk of adolescent suicide with SSRIs (R. Rubin, 2006) or ADHD drugs raising cardiovascular risk may well depress use of those medications (Nissen, 2006). While these risk scares can increase resistance to medicalization, examples suggest that by themselves they are unlikely to be a permanent source of resistance.

The one additional source of resistance is the insurance and managed-care industries. Their resistance takes the form of not covering or reimbursing certain disorders or treatments or limiting treatments to a particular age or otherwise restricting access. But this is not so much resistance to medicalization as it is part of a strategy for reducing insurance coverage or medical costs. This type of resistance is not ideological but is based on definitions of medical necessity or some kind of cost/benefit ratio. The example of obesity is instructive. For decades bariatric surgery for obesity was not covered by insurers, but in recent years it has increasingly been covered. Interventions such as gastric bypass surgery have become a growth industry in the medical world (Salant and Santry, 2006). To my knowledge, no one has yet researched the impact of health insurance on specific medicalized categories, but it seems clear that insurance can both promote and limit medicalization.

It is worth restating that one reason for medicalization in our society is related to the way in which we finance human services. The only way individuals can get the services they want or need to be paid for is to define them as medical problems. Thus, there is an incentive to define problems as medical so that their treatment can be reimbursed by health insurance. This obviously encourages increased medicalization. Health spending now constitutes 16 percent of the nation's gross domestic product (Pear, 2006). While it is difficult to assess what percentage of this spending is related to medicalization, it is possible that sometime in the future an assessment will conclude that medicalization has unnecessarily increased our medical costs and should somehow be reduced. Such financial resistance is imaginable but is not on the horizon at the moment.

In rare situations there can be medical interventions without medicalization. While this is not actually a form of active resistance to medicalization, it does provide an alternative model for medical involvement. Domestic violence is the best example of this. For nearly two decades physicians have been involved with addressing domestic violence, especially in terms of identification and prevention (Alpert, 1995). But domestic violence has not become an overriding clinical category such as "battered child syndrome" with child abuse (Conrad and Schneider, 1992; Warshaw,

1989). With domestic violence, the dominant approach has been through public health rather than the clinical setting (Flitcraft, 1997). While there have been some campaigns in recent years to talk with women in a clinical setting about domestic violence, the goal has been prevention rather than individual diagnosis. The emphasis has been to identify and protect women who are victims or survivors of domestic violence (Goldstein, 2002). The public health approach to domestic violence provides an instructive example of how physicians can intervene in serious social problems without transforming them into medicalized clinical entities.

What does this review of resistance tell us? In the sea of medicalization, there are some islands of resistance. The most successful examples of resistance, such as homosexuality and disability, politicize the issue and make it part of the agenda of a social movement. Sometimes, as with childbirth and perhaps with hospice care for dying, medicalization can be reformed so that its manifestations are no longer as extreme. There are always some groups (such as Church of Scientology or New View) that wage a battle against medicalization, but they have had relatively few successes. The Internet seems to be a potential source of resistance, although it is unlikely that the pro-ana websites will spawn many imitators. Some individuals resist medicalization of their own problems and have the resolve to seek alternative strategies for managing life difficulties. Finally, as we saw in chapter 6, risk scares about hormone replacement therapy and silicone breast implants could temporarily, at least, reduce the amount of medicalization; they didn't reduce the medicalized definitions of problems. Thus, although medicalization is not destined, it is a ubiquitous and powerful force in defining human problems.

FRONTIERS OF MEDICALIZATION

As we stand in the early twenty-first century, we can see new frontiers of medicalization. Most of these are extensions of the trends in medicalization of the past three decades, although some are only now emerging. I point to these not so much as a prediction of the future but rather as a guide to possible avenues of medicalization in the forthcoming decades.

In the wake of the Human Genome Project, it seems likely that there will be increasing claims about genetics and medical disorders. Geneticization does not automatically produce medicalization. As noted in chapter 5, the mere claim of discovering the so-called gay gene did not have much impact on the demedicalization of homosexuality. But in other cases, the impact might be different. For example, if some apparently valid genetic associations were discovered for obesity, addictions, or a propensity to violence, these discoveries might increase the medicalization of these problems. A genetic discovery in itself will not lead to medicalization but rather will affect how a condition is interpreted and promoted in the medical and social worlds. I have outlined these issues in more detail elsewhere (Conrad, 2000).

Genetics may affect medicalization in other ways. At the moment there are no genetic enhancements, but it is my firm belief that such enhancements will emerge within the next few decades. While most genetic traits are complex and would not be easily manipulated, it is certainly possible that some forms of prenatal genetic intervention could become an option. If this occurs, we may well see new traits defined as medical problems and the seeking of medicogenetic solutions. For example, if genes regulating height were located and some type of genetic engineering were developed to splice in new genes, we might see the emergence of a new "height insufficiency disorder" that prompted genetic treatment or genetic interventions to increase (or decrease) height simply according to parental preferences.

We are already witnessing a great increase in pharmaceutical intervention for human problems. The growth of retail drug sales soared from 1994 to 2004, although this escalation may be slowing down (Pear, 2006), in part because a number of drugs have been shown to carry great risks (e.g., the arthritis drug Vioxx, SSRIs for children and adolescents). But with the emergence of direct-to-consumer advertising, pharmaceutical companies can more directly define problems as illnesses and promote their own drugs as the proper solutions. Unless there is a change in the FDA regulations, it seems likely that DTC advertising will play a strong role in creating markets for drugs and expanding medicalized definitions. One could imagine, for instance, a new drug that enhances memory abilities and a new disorder, "memory deficit disorder," promoted by the pharmaceutical manufacturer. DTC advertising of both enhancements and treatments would significantly increase medicalization.

What has been termed "antiaging medicine" has seen burgeoning growth in recent years. While not surprising, given the aging baby boomers, the youth culture emphasis in American society, and the huge percentage of health care dollars spent on older people, this trend may shape our views and treatment of aging. While aging has already to a degree been medicalized, the antiaging-medicine movement redefines nearly all of aging as appropriate for medical intervention. It no longer matters whether aging is natural or not or whether one is sick or well, but only whether aspects of aging can be targets of medical intervention (Mykytyn, 2006). Aging is thus not inevitable and can be treated by medicine. This takes some of the suppositions of cosmetic surgery and transplants them to workings of the aging body. Numerous Internet sites and clinics specializing in antiaging medicine and promoting their services already exist. These may be just the leading edge of entrepreneurial medicine, with more segmented medical markets to follow.

Sociologists have pointed out that we are increasingly living in a risk society and that more and more medical risks (Lupton, 1993; Kenen, 1996) are being identified, which is leading to a medicalization of risk (Klawiter, 1998). With the increased technological capacity to assess potential "risk factors" for diseases and disorders at earlier stages, the concepts of illness and risk are becoming blurred. Medical measures such as high blood pressure, elevated cholesterol, or excessive weight are seen as risk factors for stroke, heart disease, and diabetes. But increasingly these risk factors are themselves seen as "protodisease" (Rosenberg, 2000); here risk is treated not as some statistical potential for the future but as a near-disease state. Risk means the potential for disease, but it is increasingly treated as if it were an illness in and of itself. David Greaves suggests that medicine is now treating those at risk as partial patients, people who "do not feel themselves to be ill or disabled . . . but have been informed medically [that] because they have certain characteristics, they . . . are at risk of acquiring such a disease or medical condition" (2000: 23). They may not have any symptoms, but their condition is still medicalized. The pharmaceutical industry has promoted the treatment of such risks, especially for hypertension or high cholesterol, and often with an attendant contest over the proper thresholds for risk and treatment (Wilson, 2005). Using the case of tamoxifen and breast cancer, Maren Klawiter (1998) shows how the pharmaceutical industry, the research medical community, and drug regulatory agencies operated together to reconstitute healthy women as risk subjects. While interventions for genetic risk (or susceptibility) are still mostly in the future, it seems certain that genetic risk will frequently become medical risk as well (Holtzman and Marteau, 2000). It seems likely that there will be an increased medicalization of risk, with more screening and monitoring of bodies and bodily functions. Given the incentives to locate and treat risk, these "protodiseases" are likely to expand. Thus, potentially everyone can become an object of medical attention, and the last well person will disappear (Meador, 1994).

A final frontier of medicalization is the international sphere. Medicalization has predominantly centered in the United States, and to a lesser degree in Western democracies, but with the continued spread and hegemony of Western biomedicine, the rise of the Internet, and the promise of multinational marketing, one can expect medicalized definitions and treatments to migrate to other countries (e.g., Lakoff, 2005; Castro-Vázquez, 2006, Wojnowski, 2006). But as Margaret Lock reminds us, "a huge proportion of the world's population effectively remains out of the reach of biomedicine" (2004: 123), which means they are excluded from much-needed health care as well as from much medicalization. The diffusion of medicalization will be uneven, owing to cultural resistance as well as financial barriers;

nonetheless it seems likely that in the ensuing decades medicalization will become increasingly a global phenomenon.

It is hard to imagine a world in which medicalization diminishes. Whatever the medical and social consequences, medicalization will remain a dominant approach for an increasing range of human problems. The questions remain: How will medicalization affect the organization of society, and how will we deal with the consequences?

Notes

CHAPTER 1: MEDICALIZATION

1. Several paragraphs in this section were revised from Conrad (2000).

2. According to the DSM, the diagnostic criteria for SAD include a marked and persistent fear of social or performance situations in which embarrassment may occur, an immediate anxiety response, a recognition that the fear is excessive or unreasonable, avoidance of the situation or endurance with dread, interference with daily routine or marked distress about the phobia, and the fear not being due to substance effects or other conditions (APA, 1994: 411).

CHAPTER 2: EXTENSION

1. Indeed, this understanding is gaining recognition in the literature. Riska, writing two decades after Riessman, highlights the gendered nature of the medicalization thesis by examining type A behavioral patterns as risk factors for heart disease. She writes that "the original theory on Type A personality pointed indirectly to traditional masculinity as a risk factor" (2003: 75), suggesting that certain male-specific traits have come under medical jurisdiction.

2. The efficacy of testosterone replacement therapy is not well known, although a few small studies suggest some benefit for various age-related conditions. One study suggests that testosterone decreases LDL cholesterol in older men and may improve the quality of life in men with angina, or chronic chest pain (Morley and Perry, 2003). One of the main health concerns among the aging population is frailty caused by sarcopenia, or a deterioration of lean muscle mass. Bodily frailty leaves the elderly population more prone to falls and broken bones. There is evidence that testosterone replacement therapy may increase lean muscle mass if accompanied by rehabilitation. As Morley and Perry write, "Well-designed large clinical trials in sarcopenia and/or frail men are essential to determine whether this potential is a reality or merely a modern urban myth" (p. 371).

While a small amount of clinical data suggests that testosterone therapy may have some benefit in terms of various bodily conditions later in life, it does not appear as if testosterone replacement therapy can completely reinvigorate aging male bodies. In short, testosterone replacement therapy has not yet demonstrated efficacy in reversing or correcting signs of the aging process (Wespes and Schulman, 2002).

3. Klinefelter syndrome is one of the more common developmental disorders of the reproductive tract in which a male has a chromosomal abnormality (XXY), undeveloped testes, and gynecomastia (excessive development of the mammary glands). Testosterone supplementation is often prescribed to individuals who have Klinefelter syndrome.

4. As a topical solution, Rogaine is applied to the scalp twice a day. In clinical trials, Rogaine was moderately effective, although it could only be used in men with hair loss of a certain severity.

CHAPTER 3: EXPANSION

1. More recently, Best (1999) has drawn on the work of Stallings (1990) to make a distinction between "domain expansion" and "domain elaboration." Domain elaboration is a process related to domain expansion in that it "involves the identification of new aspects of a problem" (Best, 1999: 169). These terms overlap considerably in their meaning, and both refer to the way in which expanding categories of social problem result in additional claims-makers and advocates who identify with the problem, promote its continued existence, and keep the problem alive in the public eye. To maintain consistency throughout this chapter, we have chosen to use the more familiar term "domain expansion."

2. A study by Leffers (1997) focuses on how individuals with ADHD come to understand their problems and how the social construction of the disorder affects this understanding. This chapter is more of a sociological account of the expansion of the ADHD diagnosis to adults.

3. For example, although the cohort continued to exhibit signs of hyperactivity, a twenty-year follow-up found 36 percent of the cohort symptomatic—a less widely reported statistic (e.g., *Newsweek*, 1990). Even "experts" (such as Edward Hallowell) are cited in the popular literature as saying that "seventy percent of the kids who have it continue to suffer symptoms as adults" (Stich, 1993: 77). The figure of 70 percent appears to come from a study published by Wender in 1995 but is not the most accepted estimate of persistence of symptoms.

4. DSM-III, the third revision, aimed for more rigorous diagnoses. It represented the dominance of the biopsychiatric viewpoint in psychiatry over other perspectives (Cooksey and Brown, 1998).

5. Referencing the work of others, Zametkin et al. (1990: 1361) noted that "the disorder is probably inherited in certain families" and "symptoms persist into adulthood in 40 to 60 percent of the persons with childhood hyperactivity," but these claims were made primarily in the context of justifying using an adult sample.

6. The follow-up studies using adolescent populations produced varied results (e.g., Zametkin et al., 1993; Ernst et al., 1994; Ernst et al., 1997). Additionally, with more evidence in, scientists are less sure that PET scans establish a clear marker of ADHD—in children or in adults.

7. Questions include "Do you change the radio station in your car frequently?" and "Are you always on the go, even when you don't really want to be?" The authors provide no normative standards against which to judge the answers.

8. As a claims-maker, CHADD spans several significant sectors. CHADD is buttressed by both the academic and business sectors of the ADHD community. The board of directors of CHADD includes well-known academic researchers and physicians who work in the area of ADHD.

9. Production rates do not tell the entire story: while not all of the methylphenidate production is consumed in this country, a sizable portion is. According to the United Nations 1993 statistics, the United States produces and consumes more than 80 percent of all methylphenidate (Guistolise, 1998), but the DEA has estimated that the United States consumes more than 90 percent of the 8.5 tons produced worldwide (Livingston, 1997).

10. For many years Ciba-Geigy actively proclaimed the benefits of Ritalin in advertisements. It is interesting that we have been unable to locate drug advertising for Ritalin for ADHD adults in major psychiatric or medical journals. Either Ciba-Geigy advertises Ritalin for ADHD through other channels (e.g., "detail" representatives who call on physicians or through conferences) or it has not promoted Ritalin for adult ADHD. Given the potential market, this limitation is likely because it has not been FDA approved for adult ADHD.

11. In keeping with the approach begun with DSM-III, however, such markers are not seen as establishing the etiology of the disorder; rather, they are diagnostic in nature. While the manual asserted that no biologic markers currently exist ("There are no laboratory tests that have been established as diagnostic"), through the absence of such markers, the manual gives credibility to such tests. Therefore, in refuting the absence of any such tests, the manual may have laid the groundwork for the next version of the DSM to consider laboratory tests such as PET or SPECT (single photon emission computed tomography). In fact, lay as well as professional claims-makers have been asserting the presence of genetic (as well as other biologic) markers of ADHD.

12. A recent article reported a sharp increase in the use of Ritalin among 2- to 4-year-old children enrolled in two Medicaid programs (Zito et al., 2000). While safety as well as efficacy for such young children is unknown, and diagnostic validity is even more problematic, this finding suggests that ADHD may be expanding in two directions age-wise, creating a lifelong disorder.

13. In a different domain, the medicalization of childbirth has been the gateway to the medicalization of infertility, pregnancy, and the postnatal period. It also has contributed to the medicalization of sexuality and sexual dysfunction.

CHAPTER 4: ENHANCEMENT

1. Professional medicine has long approved of off-label uses of drugs. In 1999 the American Medical Association approved a position statement (Resolution 528), introduced by the Society of Cardiovascular and Interventional Radiology, on the off-label use of devices and medications. In summary, the AMA permits physicians to decide what to prescribe for their patients and for what medical conditions, basing their decisions on "current clinical standards and not just FDA-approved indications."

2. A parallel investigation regarding "kickbacks" to doctors who allegedly prescribed Protropin was dropped, while the off-label investigations continued.

3. Poor nutrition can also stunt growth. A study in Tibet found a stunting of growth due to severe malnutrition. The researchers found this stunting to be related to other adverse consequences such as decreased intelligence, poor academic performance, and impaired development. Malnutrition kept children from reaching their genetic potential (N. Harris et al., 2001). Cases like this demonstrate the debilitating potential of malnutrition, with height as a good measure, but do not suggest that shortness causes the other dysfunctions.

4. This is an extrapolation. In 1994 about 7,000 children were believed to have short stature due to hGH deficiency, but 20,000 children were treated with hGH (*Biotechnology Business News*, 1994). Therefore, at least 13,000 children with ISS were treated that year. More recent treatment figures are difficult to estimate.

5. In sports we have the additional fairness issue of comparability of records and achievements. As I write, the issue of Barry Bonds's steroid use and its role in his surpassing of Hank Aaron's lifetime home run record is a major controversy in Major League Baseball.

6. For further discussions, see Rothman and Rothman (2003: 168–207) and Hoberman (2005: 179–213).

CHAPTER 6: MEASURING MEDICALIZATION

1. I thank Cheryl Stults, who did most of the research reported in this section.

2. In this chapter I use "HRT" to denote both estrogen replacement therapy and hormone replacement therapy, which, while they have some differences, are both examples of hormone treatment for postmenopausal women. I use the term "ERT" only where it was used in the original.

3. Most of the data in this section are drawn from research conducted with Cindy Parks Thomas, Elizabeth Goodman, and Rosemary Casler (Thomas et al., 2006). I thank these colleagues.

4. This section benefited greatly from discussions with Allan Horwitz and Jerome Wakefield.

5. Recent estimates from the National Comorbidity Survey Replication claim a 7.3 percent lifetime prevalence of "intermittent explosive disorder" (IED); the claim is that IED affects 16 million people (Kessler et al., 2006b). This represents a medicalization of having a "bad temper"—surely a problem, but is it a medical disorder?

CHAPTER 7: THE SHIFTING ENGINES
OF MEDICALIZATION

1. I contend that the consumer orientation toward medical care has expanded, subsuming or reorienting some of the social movements promoting medicalization. Moreover, there is an increasing amount of public and media promotion of health care products, procedures, and services that further spurs medicalization (including medications, surgical procedures, and other treatments). These are aimed at individuals, not as patients but as consumers.

2. Joseph E. Davis (2006) argues that the study of medicalization has become too broad in focus and should confine its analytical purview to what physicians and the medical profession do to expand medical jurisdiction. I don't believe such a constricted understanding of medicalization would do justice to this complex phenomenon.

3. Richard Smith, former editor of the *British Medical Journal*, argues that even peer-reviewed medical journals have become an extension of the marketing arm of pharmaceutical companies (R. Smith, 2005).

CHAPTER 8: MEDICALIZATION AND
ITS DISCONTENTS

1. Ellie Lee (2003) presents an interesting case in her analysis of the resistance to the medicalization of "post-abortion syndrome." She shows that both the politicized nature of abortion and a lack of scientific evidence have undermined support for this diagnosis.

References

AACE (American Association of Clinical Endocrinologists). 2002. "Medical Guidelines for Clinical Practice for the Evaluation and Treatment of Hypogonadism in Adult Male Patients." *Endocrine Practice* 8: 439–56.

Abelson, Phillip, and Donald Kennedy. 2004. "The Obesity Epidemic." *Science* 304: 1413.

Abramson, P. 1985. "Genentech's Drug Problem: Marketing Protropin." *Newsweek* 106: 70.

AFX News. 1996. "Ciba-Geigy 'Surprised' by INCB Criticism of Ritalin." February 29.

Allen, Laura S., and Roger A Gorski. 1992. "Sexual Orientation and the Size of the Human Brain." *Proceedings of the National Academy of Sciences* 89: 7199–7202.

Alpert, Elaine J. 1995. "Violence and Intimate Relationships and the Practicing Internist: New 'Disease' or New Agenda." *Annals of Internal Medicine* 123: 774–81.

AMA Science News. 2004. "New Analysis Cites Economic Impact of ADHD." September 9. www.eurekalert.org/pub_releases/2004-09/ama-nac090304.php.

Amoroso, M. 1999. "Tall Order to Weigh for Kids." *Record*, March 25, H01.

Angell, Marcia. 2003. *The Truth about Drug Companies: How They Deceive Us and What to Do about It.* New York: Random House

Angier, Natalie. 1990. "Human Growth Hormone Reverses Effects of Aging." *New York Times*, July 5, A1.

Anspach, Renee. 2003. "Gender and Health Care." Unpublished manuscript, Department of Sociology, University of Michigan, Ann Arbor.

APA (American Psychiatric Association). 1952. *Diagnostic and Statistical Manual: Mental Disorders.* Washington, D.C.: APA.

———. 1968. *Diagnostic and Statistical Manual of Mental Disorders*, 2nd ed. (DSM-II). Washington, D.C.: APA.

———. 1980. *Diagnostic and Statistical Manual of Mental Disorders*, 3rd ed. (DSM-III). Washington, D.C.: APA.

———. 1987. *Diagnostic and Statistical Manual of Mental Disorders*, 3rd ed., revised (DSM-III-R). Washington, D.C.: APA.

———. 1994. *Diagnostic and Statistical Manual of Mental Disorders*, 4th ed. (DSM-IV). Washington, D.C.: APA.

———. 2000. *Diagnostic and Statistical Manual of Mental Disorders*, 4th ed., text revision (DSM-IV-TR). Washington, D.C.: APA.

Aparasu, Rajender R., Jane R. Mort, and Anuradha Aparasu. 2001. "Inappropriate Psychotropic Agents for the Elderly." *Geriatric Times* 2 (2). www.geriatrictimes.com/g010321.html.

Appleton, Lynn M. 1995. "Rethinking Medicalization: Alcoholism and Anomalies." Pp. 59–80 in Joel Best (ed.), *Images of Issues*, 2nd ed. New York: Aldine de Gruyter.

Armstrong, David. 1995. "The Rise of Surveillance Medicine." *Sociology of Health and Illness* 17: 393–404.

Armstrong, Elizabeth. 2003. *Conceiving Risk, Bearing Responsibility: Fetal Alcohol Syndrome and the Diagnosis of Moral Disorder*. Baltimore: Johns Hopkins University Press.

Arnst, Catherine. 1999. "Attention Deficit: Is It in the Genes?" *Business Week*, November 22, 70.

Aronowitz, Robert A. 1998. *Making Sense of Illness: Science, Society and Disease*. Cambridge, UK: Cambridge University Press.

ASAPS (American Society for Aesthetic Plastic Surgery). 2004. "11.9 Million Cosmetic Procedures in 2004." www.surgery.org/press/news-release.php?iid=395.

———. 2005a. "Highlights of the ASAPS 2005 Statistics on Cosmetic Surgery." www.surgery.org/press/procedurefacts-asqf.php.

———. 2005b. "Statistics 2005." www.surgery.org/press/statistics-2005.php.

Auerbach, S. 1996. "Is Human Growth Overprescribed? Many Short Children Are Taking It without a Medical Reason, Study Finds." *Washington Post*, August 27, Z07.

Bailey, J. Michael, and Richard C. Pillard. 1991. "A Genetic Study of Male Sexual Orientation." *Archives of General Psychiatry* 48: 1089–96.

Bailey, J. Michael, R. C. Pillard, M. C. Neale, and Y. Agyei. 1993. "Heritable Factors Influence Sexual Orientation in Women." *Archives of General Psychiatry* 50: 217–23.

Balint, Michael. 1957. *The Doctor, His Patient, and the Illness*. New York: International Universities Press.

Ballard, Karen, and Mary Ann Elston. 2005. "Medicalization: A Multi-Dimensional Concept." *Social Theory and Health* 3: 228–41.

Ballard, Shirley, Morna Bolan, Michael Burton, et al. 1997. "The Neurological Basis of Attention Deficit Hyperactivity Disorder." *Adolescence* 32 (128): 855–62.

Barker, Kristin K. 2002. "Self-Help Literature and the Making of an Illness Identity: The Case of Fibromyalgia Syndrome (FMS)." *Social Problems* 49: 279–300.

———. 2005a. "Electronic Support Groups and Contested Chronic Illness: An Exploration of Electronic Ethnography." Paper presented at the "Contours of Contestation" conference, University of Victoria.

———. 2005b. *The Fibromyalgia Story: Medical Authority and Women's Worlds of Pain*. Philadelphia: Temple University Press.

Barkley, Russell A. 1997. *ADHD and the Nature of Self-Control*. New York: Guilford.

Barkley, Russell A., and Joseph Biederman. 1997. "Toward a Broader Definition of the Age-of-Onset Criterion for Attention-Deficit Hyperactivity Disorder." *Journal of the American Academy of Child and Adolescent Psychiatry* 36: 1204–10.

Barlas, Stephen. 2005. "Special Education Bill Limits Use of Stimulants." *Washington Post*, February 1, 10.

Barry, Ellen. 2002. "Mass. Group Sues Paxil Drugmaker." *Boston Globe*, October 26, A3.

Barsky, Arthur J., and Jonathan F. Boros. 1995. "Somatization and Medicalization in the Era of Managed Care." *Journal of the American Medical Association* 274: 1931–34.

Bartholomew, Robert E. 2000. *Exotic Deviance: Medicalizing Cultural Idioms from Strangeness to Illness*. Boulder: University Press of Colorado.

Bartlett, K. 1990. "Attention Deficit: Scientists Move toward Understanding of Brain Disorder Once Thought Limited to Children." *Houston Chronicle*, December 2, 6G.

Batavia, Andrew I., and Kay Schriner. 2001. "The Americans with Disabilities Act as Engine of Social Change: Models of Disability and the Potential of a Civil Rights Approach." *Policy Studies Journal* 29: 690–702.

Bayer, Ronald. 1985. "AIDS and the Gay Community: Between the Specter and the Promise of Medicine." *Social Research* 52 (3): 581–606.

———. 1987. *Homosexuality and American Psychiatry: The Politics of Diagnosis.* Princeton: Princeton University Press.

Becker, Gay, and R. Nachtigall. 1992. "Eager for Medicalization: The Social Production of Infertility as a Disease." *Sociology of Health and Illness* 14: 456–71.

Bell, Susan E. 1987. "Changing Ideas: The Medicalization of Menopause." *Social Science and Medicine* 24: 535–42.

———. 1990. "Sociological Perspectives on the Medicalization of Menopause." *Annals of New York Academy of Sciences* 592: 173–78.

Bercu, B. B. 1996. "The Growth Conundrum: Growth Hormone Treatment of the Nongrowth Hormone Deficient Child." Editorial. *Journal of the American Medical Association* 276: 567–68.

Berenson, Alex. 2005. "Sales of Impotence Drugs Fall, Defying Expectations." *New York Times*, December 4, 1.

Bergler, Edmund. 1956. *Homosexuality: Disease or Way of Life?* New York: Hill and Wang.

Best, Joel. 1990. *Threatened Children: Rhetoric and Concern about Child Victims.* Chicago: University of Chicago Press.

———. 1999. *Random Violence: How We Talk about New Crimes and New Victims.* Berkeley: University of California Press.

Bieber, Irving, et al. 1962. *Homosexuality: A Psychoanalytic Study.* New York: Basic Books.

Biederman, Joseph, Stephen Farone, Sharon Milberger, et al. 1996. "A Prospective Four-Year Follow-up Study of Attention-Deficit Hyperactivity and Related Disorders." *Archives of General Psychiatry* 53: 137–46.

Biotechnology Business News. 1994. "Efficacy of Growth Hormones Questioned in US." October 24.

Blum, Linda M., and Nena F. Stracuzzi. 2004. "Gender in the Prozac Nation. Popular Discourse and Productive Femininity." *Gender and Society* 18 (3): 269–86.

Bond, John. 1992. "The Medicalization of Dementia." *Journal of Aging Studies* 6: 397–403.

Bouhanna, P., and J. C. Dardour. 2000. *Hair Replacement Surgery: Textbook and Atlas.* New York: Springer.

Bowles, Samuel, Herbert Gintis, and M. Osborne. 2001. "The Determinants of Earnings: A Behavioral Approach." *Journal of Economic Literature* 39: 1137–76.

Bradley, C. A., and T. M. Sodeman. 1990. "Human Growth Hormone: Its Use and Abuse." *Clinics in Laboratory Medicine* 10: 473–77.

Bradley, Susan, et al. 1991. "Interim Report of the DSM-IV Subcommittee on Gender Identity Disorders." *Archives of Sexual Behavior* 20 (4): 333–43.

Breggin, Peter. 1998. *Talking Back to Ritalin.* Monroe, ME: Common Courage.

British Medical Journal. 2002. Special issue on medicalization. 234 (7342): 859–926.

Bromfield, Richard. 1996. "Fad or Disorder?" *American Health*, June, 32.

Broom, Dorothy H., and Roslyn V. Woodward. 1996. "Medicalization Reconsidered: Toward a Collaborative Approach to Care." *Sociology of Health and Illness* 18: 357–78.

Brown, Phil. 1995. "Naming and Framing: The Social Construction of Diagnosis and Illness." In Phil Brown (ed.), *Perspectives in Medical Sociology*, 3rd ed. Prospect Heights, IL: Waveland.

Brumberg, Joan Jacobs. 1988. *Fasting Girls.* New York: Random House.

———. 2001. "Anorexia Nervosa in Context." Pp. 94–108 in Peter Conrad (ed.), *The Sociology of Health and Illness: Critical Perspectives*, 6th ed. New York: Worth.

Buchanan, Allen, Dan Brock, Norman Daniels, and Daniel Wikler. 2000. *From Chance to Choice: Genetics and Justice*. New York: Cambridge University Press.

Bury, Michael. 1986. "Social Constructionism and the Development of Medical Sociology." *Sociology of Health and Illness* 8: 137–69.

———. 2005. *Health and Illness*. Cambridge, UK: Polity.

Busschbach, J., P. von Horikx, J. van den Bosch, et al. 1999. "The Psychosocial Functioning of Children with Short Stature: The Role of Recognition." In U. Eiholzer, F. Haverkamp, and L. Voss (eds.), *Growth, Stature, and Psychosocial Well-Being*. Seattle: Hogrefe and Huber.

Butler, R. N., M. Fossel, S. Mitchell, et al. 2000. "Anti-Aging Medicine: Efficacy and Safety of Hormones and Antioxidants." *Geriatrics* 55: 48–58.

Campbell, Harvey. 1983. "A Sexual Minority: Homosexuality and Mental Health Care." *American Journal of Social Psychiatry* 2: 26–35.

Cantwell, Dennis P. 1975. "Psychiatric Illness in the Families of Hyperactive Children." *Archives of General Psychiatry* 27: 414–17.

Caplan, Paula J. 1995. *They Say You're Crazy: How the World's Most Powerful Psychiatrists Decide Who's Normal*. Reading, MA: Addison-Wesley.

Carpiano, Richard M. 2001. "Passive Medicalization: The Case of Viagra and Erectile Dysfunction." *Sociological Spectrum* 21: 441–50.

Caspi, Avshalom, Karen Sugden, Terrie Moffit, et al. 2003. "Influence of Life Stress on Depression: Moderation by a Polymorphism in the 5-HTT Gene." *Science* 301: 386–89.

Castro-Vázquez, Genaro. 2006. "The Politics of Viagra: Gender, Dysfunction, and Reproduction in Japan." *Body and Society* 12: 109–29.

CDC (Centers for Disease Control). 2002. "New CDC Report Looks at Attention Deficit/Hyperactivity Disorder." www.cdc.gov/nchs/pressroom/02news/attendefic.htm.

Clarke, Adele E., Laura Mamo, Jennifer Fosket, et al. 2006. *Biomedicalization: Technoscience, Health, and Illness in the U.S.* Durham, NC: Duke University Press.

Clarke, Adele E., Janet K. Shim, Laura Mamo, et al. 2003. "Biomedicalization: Technoscientific Transformations of Health, Illness, and U.S. Biomedicine." *American Sociological Review* 68: 161–94.

Cohler, Bertram, and Robert Galatzer-Levy. 2000. *The Course of Gay and Lesbian Lives*. Chicago: University of Chicago Press.

Conrad, Peter. 1975. "The Discovery of Hyperkinesis: Notes on the Medicalization of Deviant Behavior." *Social Problems* 23: 12–21.

———. 1976. *Identifying Hyperactive Children: The Medicalization of Deviant Behavior*. Lexington, MA: D. C. Heath.

———. 1979. "Types of Medical Social Control." *Sociology of Health and Illness* 1: 1–11.

———. 1986. "The Social Meaning of AIDS." *Social Policy* 17 (1): 51–54.

———. 1992. "Medicalization and Social Control." *Annual Review of Sociology* 18: 209–32.

———. 1997. "Public Eyes and Private Genes: Historical Frames, News Constructions, and Social Problems." *Social Problems* 44: 139–54.

———. 1999. "A Mirage of Genes." *Sociology of Health and Illness* 21: 228–41.

———. 2000. "Medicalization, Genetics, and Human Problems." Pp. 322–33 in Chloe Bird, Peter Conrad, and Allen Fremont (eds.), *The Handbook of Medical Sociology*, 5th ed. Upper Saddle River, NJ: Prentice-Hall.

———. 2005. "The Shifting Engines of Medicalization." *Journal of Health and Social Behavior* 46: 3–14.

———. 2006. "Introduction to Expanded Edition." *Identifying Hyperactive Children: The Medicalization of Deviant Behavior.* Expanded ed. Aldershot, UK: Ashgate.

Conrad, Peter, and Allison Angell. 2004. "Homosexuality and Remedicalization." *Society* 41 (5): 32–39.

Conrad, Peter, and Heather Jacobson. 2003. "Enhancing Biology? Cosmetic Surgery and Breast Augmentation." In Simon Williams, G. A. Bendelow, and L. Birke (eds.), *Debating Biology: Sociological Reflections on Health, Medicine, and Society.* London: Routledge.

Conrad, Peter, and Valerie Leiter. 2004. "Medicalization, Markets, and Consumers." *Journal of Health and Social Behavior* 45: 158–76.

———. 2005. "From Lydia Pinkham to Queen Levitra: Direct-to-Consumer Advertising and Medicalization." Paper presented at the meetings of the American Sociological Association, Philadelphia.

Conrad, Peter, and Susan Markens. 2001. "Constructing the 'Gay Gene' in the News: Optimism and Skepticism in the US and British Press." *Health* 5: 373–400.

Conrad, Peter, and Deborah Potter. 2000. "From Hyperactive Children to ADHD Adults: Observations on the Expansion of Medical Categories." *Social Problems* 47: 59–82.

———. 2004. "Human Growth Hormone and the Temptations of Biomedical Enhancement." *Sociology of Health and Illness* 26: 184–215.

Conrad, Peter, and Joseph W. Schneider. 1980. *Deviance and Medicalization: From Badness to Sickness.* St. Louis: Mosby.

———. 1992. *Deviance and Medicalization: From Badness to Sickness.* Expanded ed. Philadelphia: Temple University Press.

Cooksey, Elizabeth, and Phil Brown. 1998. "Spinning on Its Axes: DSM and the Social Construction of Psychiatric Diagnosis." *International Journal of Health Services* 28: 525–54.

Cooper, Lesley, 1997 "Myalgic Encephalomyelitis and the Medical Encounter." *Sociology of Health and Illness* 19: 186–207.

Cooper, Wendy. 1971. *Hair: Sex, Society, Symbolism.* New York: Stein and Day.

Cooper, William O., Patrick G. Arbogast, Hua Ding, et al. 2006. "Trends in Prescribing Antipsychotic Medications to US Children." *Ambulatory Pediatrics* 6: 79–83.

Corpas, E., S. M. Harman, and M. R. Blackman. 1993. "Human Growth Hormone and Human Aging." *Endocrine Reviews* 14: 20–37.

Cowley, Geoffrey. 1996. "Attention: Aging Men." *Newsweek,* July 26, 68–75.

Cowley, Geoffrey, and Joshua Cooper Ramo. 1993. "The Not-Young and the Restless." *Newsweek,* July 26, 48–49.

Cowley, Geoffrey, and Karen Springen. 2002. "The End of the Age of Estrogen." *Newsweek,* July 22, 38.

Crary, David. 2004. "Activists Gather to Win 'Fat Acceptance.'" *Boston Globe,* August 4, A6.

Crouch, Robert A. 1997. "Letting the Deaf Be Deaf: Reconsidering the Use of Cochlear Implants in Prelingually Deaf Children." *Hastings Center Report* 27 (4): 14–21.

Curry, Timothy J., and Matthew A. Salerno. 1999. "A Comment on the Use of Anabolic Steroids in Women's Olympic Swimming." *International Review for the Sociology of Sport* 34: 173–80.

Cutler, L., J. B. Silvers, J. Singh, et al. 1996. "Short Stature and Growth Hormone Therapy: A National Study of Physician Recommendation Patterns." *Journal of the American Medical Association* 276: 531–37.

Daniels, Norman. 1994. "The Genome Project, Individual Differences, and Just Health Care." In T. F. Murphy and M. A. Lappe (eds.), *Justice and the Genome Project.* Berkeley: University of California Press.

Dawber, Rodney, and Dominique Van Neste (eds). 1995. *Hair and Scalp Disorders: Common Presenting Signs, Differential Diagnosis, and Treatment.* London: Martin Dunitz.

Davis, Joseph E. 2006. "How Medicalization Lost Its Way." *Society* 43 (6): 51–56.

DeGrandpre, Richard. 1999. *Ritalin Nation: Rapid-Fire Culture and the Transformation of Human Consciousness.* New York: Norton.

D'Emilio, John. 2002. *The World Turned: Essays on Gay History, Politics, and Culture.* Durham: Duke University Press.

Dennis, Dion. 1997. "AIDS and the New Medical Gaze: Bio-Politics, AIDS, and Homosexuality." *Journal of Homosexuality* 32 (3–4): 169–84.

Diamont, Louis. 1987. "The Therapies." Pp. 199–217 in Louis Diamont (ed.), *Male and Female Homosexuality: Psychological Approaches.* New York: Hemisphere.

Diekema, Douglas S. 1990. "Is Taller Really Better? Growth Hormone Therapy in Short Children." *Perspectives in Biology and Medicine* 34: 109–23.

Diller, Lawrence H. 1996. "The Run on Ritalin: Attention Deficit Disorder and Stimulant Treatment in the 1990s." *Hastings Center Report* 26 (2): 12–18.

———. 1997. *Running on Ritalin.* New York: Bantam Books.

Dobrin, Stanley. 1994. Testimony on behalf of Benjamin Dobrin before the House Committee on Business, Subcommittee on Regulation, Business Opportunities, and Technology, on the Questionable Practices in Drug Industry Marketing and Promotion, 12 October, 106th Cong., 1st sess.

Doctor's Guide Global Edition. 2000. "FDA Approves Prescription AndroGel for Low Testosterone." Buffalo Grove, IL: Doctor's Guide. www.pslgroup.com/dg/1780fa.htm.

Domino, Marisa Elena, David S. Salkever, D. A. Zarin, and H. A. Pincus. 1998. "The Impact of Managed Care on Psychiatry." *Administration and Policy in Mental Health* 26 (2): 149–57.

Dubos, Rene. 1959. *Mirage of Health.* New York: Harper and Row.

Durkheim, Emile. 1933. *The Division of Labor in Society.* New York: Free Press.

Dyer, Allen R. 1997. "Ethics, Advertising, and Assisted Reproduction: The Goals and Methods of Advertising." *Women's Health Issues* 7: 143–48.

Eberstadt, Mary. 1999. "Why Ritalin Rules." *Policy Review* 94. www.policyreview.com/apr99/eberstadt.html.

Economist. 2002. "Walk Tall." April 27, 8.

Elia, Josephine, Paul J. Ambrosini, and Judith L. Rapoport. 1999. "Treatment of Attention-Deficit-Hyperactivity Disorder." *New England Journal of Medicine* 340: 780–88.

Elliott, Carl. 1999. "Pursued by Happiness and Beaten Senseless: Prozac and the American Dream." *Hastings Center Report* 30 (2): 7–12.

———. 2003. *Better Than Well: American Medicine Meets the American Dream.* New York: Norton.

Engelhardt, H. Tristan. 1974. "The Disease of Masturbation: Values and the Concept of Disease." *Bulletin of the History of Medicine* 48: 234–48.

Epstein, Steven. 1988. "Moral Contagion and the Medicalizing of Gay Identity." *Research in Law, Deviance, and Social Control* 9: 3–36.

———. 1996. *Impure Science: AIDS, Activism, and the Politics of Knowledge.* Berkeley: University of California Press.

———. 2003. "Sexualizing Governance and Medicalizing Identities: The Emergence of 'State-Centered' LGBT Health Politics in the United States." *Sexualities* 6: 131–71.

Erchak, Gerald M., and Richard Rosenfeld. 1989. "Learning Disabilities, Dyslexia, and the Medicalization of the Classroom." In Joel Best (ed.), *Images of Issues*. New York: Aldine de Gruyter.

Erickson, Deborah. 1990. "Big-Time Orphan: Human Growth Hormone Could Be a Blockbuster." *Scientific American*, September, 164–65.

Ernst, Monique, Robert M. Cohen, et al. 1997. "Cerebral Glucose Metabolism in Adolescent Girls with Attention-Deficit/Hyperactivity Disorder." *Journal of the American Academy of Child and Adolescent Psychiatry* 36: 1399–1406.

Ernst, Monique, Laura L. Lievenauer, et al. 1994. "Reduce Brain Metabolism in Hyperactive Girls." *Journal of the American Academy of Child and Adolescent Psychiatry* 33: 858–68.

Escoffier, Jeffrey. 1998–99. "The Invention of Safer-Sex." *Berkeley Journal of Sociology* 43: 1–30.

Estes, Carroll L., and E. A. Binney. 1989. "The Biomedicalization of Aging: Dangers and Dilemmas." *Gerontologist* 29: 587–96.

Fabbri, A., A. Aversa, and A. Isidori. 1997. "Erectile Dysfunction: An Overview." *Human Reproduction Update* 3: 455–66.

Fackelmann, Kathy. 1990. "Hormone May Restore Muscle in Elderly. Research by Daniel Rudman." *Science News* 138: 23.

Fainaru-Wada, Mark, and Lance Williams. 2006. *Game of Shadows: Barry Bonds, Balco, and the Steroid Scandal That Rocked Professional Sports*. New York: Gotham Books.

Faircloth, Christopher A. 2003. *Aging Bodies: Images and Everyday Experience*. Walnut Creek, CA: AltaMira.

Faraone, Stephen V., and Joseph Beiderman. 1998. "Neurobiology of Attention-Deficit Hyperactivity Disorder." *Biology and Psychiatry* 44: 951–58.

FDA (Food and Drug Administration). 2004. "FDA Talk Paper: New Warnings for Strattera." www.fda.gov/bbs/topics/ANSWERS/2004/ANS01335.html.

Figert, Anne E. 1995. "The Three Faces of PMS: The Professional, Gendered, and Scientific Structuring of a Psychiatric Disorder." *Social Problems* 42: 56–73.

Fischer, David. 1997. "The Bald Truth: Americans Turn to Weaves, Rugs, Plugs, and Drugs to Alleviate Hair Loss." *U.S. News and World Report*, August 4, 44.

Flitcraft, Anne. 1997. "Learning from the Paradoxes of Domestic Violence." *Journal of the American Medical Association* 277: 1400–1401.

Ford, W. E. 1998. "Medical Necessity: Its Impact in Managed Mental Health Care." *Psychiatric Services* 49: 183–84.

Foreman, Judy. 1992. "Scientists Are Seeking Keys to How the Body Ages." *Boston Globe*, September 28, 38.

———. 2005. "Antiaging Drug Falls Short of Hype." *Boston Globe*, October 31, C1.

Foucault, Michel. 1965. *Madness and Civilization*. New York: Random House.

———. 1966. *Birth of the Clinic*. New York: Vintage.

Fox, Nick, Katie Ward, and Alan O'Rourke. 2005. "Pro-Anorexia, Weight-Loss Drugs, and the Internet: An 'Anti-Recovery' Explanatory Model of Anorexia." *Sociology of Health and Illness* 27: 944–71.

Fox, Patrick. 1989. "From Senility to Alzheimer's Disease: The Rise of the Alzheimer's Movement." *Milbank Quarterly* 67: 58–101.

Fox, Renee C. 1977. "The Medicalization and Demedicalization of American Society." *Daedalus* 106: 9–22.

Frankford, David M. 1998. "The Treatment/Enhancement Distinction as an Armament in the Policy Wars." In Erik Parens (ed.), *Enhancing Human Traits: Ethical and Social Implications.* Washington, D.C.: Georgetown University Press.

Freidson, Eliot. 1970. *Profession of Medicine.* New York: Dodd, Mead.

Freudenheim, Milt. 2004. "Behavior Drugs Lead in Sales for Children." *New York Times,* May 17, A9.

———. 2005. "Insurers Balk at Bariatric Operations, Citing Cost and Risks." *New York Times,* May 27, C1.

Friedan, Betty. 1993. *The Fountain of Age.* New York: Simon and Schuster.

Friedman, David. 2001. *A Mind of Its Own: A Cultural History of the Penis.* New York: Free Press.

Frieze, Irene H., Josephine Olson, and Deborah C. Good. 1990. "Perceived and Actual Discrimination in the Salaries of Male and Female Managers." *Journal of Applied Social Psychology* 20: 46–67.

Fukuyama, Francis. 2002. *Our Posthuman Future: Consequences of the Biotechnology Revolution.* New York: Picador.

Furedi, Frank. 2006. "The End of Professional Dominance." *Society* 43 (6): 14–18.

Gallagher, Eugene B., and C. Kristina Sionean. 2004. "Where Medicalization Boulevard Meets Commercialization Alley." *Journal of Policy Studies* 16: 3–62.

Gallup Organization. 2001. Gallup poll as cited in www.religioustolerance.org/hom_poll2.htm.

Gardiner, Harris. 2005. "Use of Attention Deficit Disorder Drugs Found to Soar among Adults." *New York Times,* September 15.

Gatens, Moira. 1996. *Imaginary Bodies: Ethics, Power, and Corporeality.* New York: Routledge.

Geller, Adam. 2006. "Consumers Turn to Their DNA for Answers." Associated Press, March 28.

Genentech. 1994. Written statement prepared for the House Committee on Business, Subcommittee on Regulation, Business Opportunities, and Technology, on the Questionable Practices in Drug Industry Marketing and Promotion. 12 October, 106th Cong., 1st sess.

Gimlin, Deborah. 2000. "Cosmetic Surgery: Beauty as a Commodity." *Qualitative Sociology* 23: 77–98.

Gittleman, Rachel, Salvatore Mannuzza, Ronald Shenker, and Noreen Bonagura. 1985. "Hyperactive Boys Almost Grown Up." *Archives of General Psychiatry* 42: 937–47.

Gladwell, Malcolm. 1999. "Running from Ritalin." *New Yorker,* February 15, 80–86.

Glasbrenner, K. 1986. "Technology Spurt Resolves Growth Hormone Problem, Ends Shortage." *Journal of the American Medical Association* 255: 581–84, 587.

Goldman, Larry S., Myron Genel, Robecca J. Bezman, and Priscilla J. Slanetz. 1998. "Diagnosis and Treatment of Attention-Deficit/Hyperactivity Disorder in Children and Adults." *Journal of the American Medical Association* 279: 1100–1107.

Goldstein, Rachel Y. 2002. "Two Approaches to the Medical Treatment of Domestic Violence: An Exploration of the Clinical and Public Health Perspectives." Senior honors thesis, Department of Sociology, Brandeis University.

Goode, Erica. 2002. "Psychotherapy Shows a Rise over Decade, but Time Falls." *New York Times,* November 6, A21.

Gooren, Louis. 2003. "Androgen Deficiency in the Aging Male: Benefits and Risks of Androgen Supplementation." *Journal of Steroid Biochemistry and Molecular Biology* 85: 349–55.

Grady, Denise. 2004. "Operation for Obesity Leaves Some in Misery." *New York Times,* May 4, D1.

Grady, Denise, David Herrington, Vera Bittner, et al. 2002. "Heart and Estrogen/Progestin Replacement Study Follow-up (HERS II): Cardiovascular Outcomes during 6.8 Years of Hormone Therapy." *Journal of the American Medical Association* 288: 49–57.

Greaves, David. 2000. "The Creation of Partial Patients." *Cambridge Quarterly of Health Care Ethics* 9: 23–27.

Green, Harvey. 1986. *Fit for America: Health, Fitness, and Sport in American Society.* New York: Pantheon.

Green, Richard. 1987. *The "Sissy Boy Syndrome" and the Development of Homosexuality.* New Haven: Yale University Press.

Green, Richard, and John Money. 1960. "Incongruous Gender Role: Nongenital Manifestations in Prepubertal Boys." *Journal of Nervous and Mental Disease* 131: 160–68.

Groopman, Jerome. 2002. "Hormones for Men." *New Yorker,* July 29.

Gross, Mortimer B., and William E. Wilson. 1974. *Minimum Brain Dysfunction.* New York: Burnner Mazel.

Guadagnoli, Edward, and Patricia Ward. 1998. "Patient Participation in Decision-Making." *Social Science and Medicine* 47: 329–39.

Guistolise, Jodi. 1998. "Special Section: Attention Deficit Disorder: The Ritalin Epidemic." *Home Education* 15 (3) : 30–31.

Gullette, Margaret Morganroth. 1997. "All Together Now: The New Sexual Politics of Midlife Bodies." Pp. 221–47 in Laurence Goldstein (ed.), *The Male Body: Features, Destinies, Exposures.* Ann Arbor: University of Michigan Press.

Hacking, Ian. 1995. *Rewriting the Soul: Multiple Personality and the Sciences of Memory.* Princeton: Princeton University Press.

Hadler, Norton. 2004. *The Last Well Person: How to Stay Well Despite the Health Care System.* Montreal: McGill–Queen's University Press.

Haiken, Elizabeth. 1997. *Venus Envy. A History of Cosmetic Surgery.* Baltimore: Johns Hopkins University Press.

——. 2000. "The Making of the Modern Face: Cosmetic Surgery." *Social Research* 67: 81–97.

Haines, Herb. 1989. "Primum Non Nocere: Chemical Execution and the Limits of Medical Social Control." *Social Problems* 36: 442–54.

Hales, Dianne, and Robert E. Hales. 1993. "Pay Attention: Hyperactivity Isn't Just for Children Anymore." *American Health,* September 12, 62–65.

Hall, Stephen S. 2003. "The Quest for a Smart Pill." *Scientific American* 289 (3): 54–65.

——. 2005. "The Short of It." *New York Times Magazine,* October 16.

Halliwell, Emma, and Helga Dittmar. 2003. "A Qualitative Investigation of Women's and Men's Body Image Concerns and Their Attitudes toward Aging." *Sex Roles* 49: 675–84.

Hallowell, Edward M., and John J. Ratey. 1994. *Driven to Distraction.* New York: Pantheon Books.

Halpern, Sydney A. 1990. "Medicalization as a Professional Process: Postwar Trends in Pediatrics." *Journal of Health and Social Behavior* 31: 28–42.

Hamer, Dean, and Peter Copeland. 1994. *The Science of Sexual Desire: The Search for the Gay Gene and the Biology of Behavior.* New York: Simon and Schuster.

Hamer, Dean, Stella Hu, Victoria L. Magnuson, Nan Hu, and Angela M. L. Pattatucci. 1993. "A Linkage between DNA Markers on the X Chromosome and Male Sexual Orientation." *Science* 261: 321–27.

Hardey, Michael. 2001. "'E-Health': The Internet and the Transformation of Patients to Consumers and Producers of Health Knowledge." *Information, Communication, and Society* 4: 388–405.

Harris, David Alan. 2001. "Using B-Blockers to Control Stage Fright: A Dancer's Dilemma." *Medical Problems of Performing Artists* 16 (2): 72–76.

Harris, N. S., P. B. Crauford, P. H. Yeshe Yangzorn, et al. 2001. "Nutritional and Health Status of Tibetan Children Living at High Altitudes." *New England Journal of Medicine* 34: 341–47.

Hart, Nikki, with Noah Grand and Kevin Reilly. 2006. "Making the Grade: The Gender Gap, ADHD, and the Medicalization of Boyhood." Pp. 132–64 in Dana Rosenfeld and Christopher A. Faircloth (eds.), *Medicalized Masculinities*. Philadelphia: Temple University Press.

Hartley, Heather. 2003. "'Big Pharma' in Our Bedrooms: An Analysis of the Medicalization of Women's Sexual Problems." *Advances in Gender Research* 7: 89–129.

Hartley, Heather, and Leonore Tiefer. 2003. "Taking a Biological Turn: The Push for a 'Female Viagra' and the Medicalization of Women's Sexual Problems." *Women's Studies Quarterly* 31 (spring/summer): 42–54.

Hartmann, Thom. 1994. *Attention Deficit Disorder: A Different Perception*. New York: Underwood Books.

Hays, Jennifer, Judith K. Ockene, Robert L. Brunner, et al. 2003. "Effects of Estrogen Plus Progestin on Health-Related Quality of Life." *New England Journal of Medicine* 348 (19): 1839–54.

HealthGrades. 2005. "Rates Continue to Rise but Vary Widely by Hospital and Region." *HealthGrades Third Annual Report on "Patient-Choice" Cesarean Section Rates in the United States*. www.healthgrades.com./media/dms/pdf/PatientChoiceCSectionStudy2005Sept12.pdf.

Healthy People, 2010. 2003. www.cdc.gov/nchs/about/otheract/hpdata2010/abouthp.htm.

Healy, David. 1997. *The Antidepressant Era*. Cambridge: Harvard University Press.

Hensley, Scott. 2005. "Some Drug Makers Are Curtailing TV Ad Spending." *Wall Street Journal*, May 16.

Hepworth, Mike, and Mike Featherstone. 1998. "The Male Menopause: Lay Accounts and the Cultural Reconstruction of Midlife." Pp. 276–301 in Sarah Nettleton and Jonathan Watson (eds.), *The Body in Everyday Life*. London: Routledge.

Herek, Gregory M., and John Capitanio. 1999. "AIDS Stigma and Sexual Prejudice." *American Behavioral Scientist* 42 (7): 1126–43.

Hersh, Adam L., Marcia L. Stefanick, and Randall S. Stafford. 2004. "National Use of Postmenopausal Hormone Therapy: Annual Trends and Response to Recent Evidence." *Journal of the American Medical Association* 291 (1): 47–53.

Hilchey, T. 1994. "Hormone Helps AIDS Patients Gain Weight." *New York Times*, October 16, 30.

Hilgartner, Stephen, and Charles Bosk. 1988. "The Rise and Fall of Social Problems." *American Journal of Sociology* 94: 53–78.

Hintz, Raymond L. 1996. "Growth Hormone Treatment of Idiopathic Short Stature." *Hormone Research* 46: 208–14.

Hintz, Raymond L., K. M. Attie, J. Baptista, et al. 1999. "Effect of Growth Hormone Treatment on Adult Height of Children with Idiopathic Short Stature." *New England Journal of Medicine* 30: 502–7.

Hislop, Jenny, and Sara Arber. 2003. "Understanding Women's Sleep: Beyond Medicalization-Healthicization." *Sociology of Health and Illness* 25 (7): 815–37.

Hoberman, John. 1992. *Mortal Engines: The Science of Performance and the Dehumanization of Sport*. New York: Free Press.

———. 1995. "Listening to Steroids." *Wilson Quarterly* 19: 35–44.

———. 2005. *Testosterone Dreams: Rejuvenation, Aphrodesia, Doping.* Berkeley: University of California Press.

Holtzman, Neil A., and Theresa M. Marteau. 2000. "Will Genetics Revolutionize Medicine." *New England Journal of Medicine* 343: 141–44.

Horwitz, Allan. 2002. *Creating Mental Illness.* Chicago: University of Chicago Press.

Horwitz, Allan, and Jerome Wakefield. Forthcoming. *The Loss of Sadness: How Psychiatry Transformed Normal Misery into Depressive Disorder.* Oxford University Press.

http://usgovinfo.about.com/od/olderamericans/a/obesitypolicy.htm. "Medicare Revises Obesity Coverage Policy."

Hu, Stella, Angela M. L. Pattatucci, Chavis Peterson, et al. 1995. "Linkage between Sexual Orientation and Chromosome Xq28 in Males but Not in Females." *Nature Genetics* 11: 248–56.

Hulley, Stephen, Curt Furberg, Elizabeth Barrett-Connor, et al., for the HERS Research Group. 2002. "Noncardiovascular Disease Outcomes during 6.8 Years of Hormone Therapy: Heart and Estrogen/Progestin Replacement Study Follow-up (HERS II)." *Journal of the American Medical Association* 288: 58–64.

Illich, Ivan. 1976. *Medical Nemesis.* New York: Pantheon.

Imershein, Allen W., and Carroll L. Estes. 1996. "From Health Services to Medical Markets: The Commodity Transformation of Medical Production and the Nonprofit Sector." *International Journal of Health Services* 26: 221–38.

IMS Health. 2001. "World Pharma Sales 2001: US Still Driving Growth." www.imshealth.com/web/content/0,3148,64576068_63872702_70260998_70328515,00.html.

———. 2004. "IMS Reports 11.5 Percent Dollar Growth in U.S. Prescription Sales." www.imshealth.com/ims/portal/front/articleC/0,2777,6599_3665_44771558,00.html.

Inlander, Charles B. 1998. "Consumer Health." *Social Policy* 28 (3): 40–42.

Institute of Medicine. 2004. *Testosterone and Aging. Clinical Research Directions.* Washington, D.C.: National Academies Press.

IOC (International Olympic Committee). 2000. "Olympic Movement Anti Doping Code." www.medycynasportowa.pl/download/doping_code_e.pdf#search=%22Olympic%20Movement%20Anti-Doping%20Code%22.

Irvine, Janice. 1995. "Regulated Passions: The Invention of Inhibited Sexual Desire and Sexual Addiction." In Jennifer Terry and Jacqueline Urla (eds.), *Deviant Bodies.* Bloomington: Indiana University Press.

Irvine, Leslie. 1999. *Codependent Forevermore: The Invention of Self in a Twelve Step Group.* Chicago: University of Chicago Press.

Isay, Richard. 2002. "Remove Gender Identity Disorder from DSM." *Pediatric News.* www.psych.org/pnews/97-11-21/isay.html.

Jacobson, Nora. 2000. *Cleavage: Technology, Controversy, and the Ironies of the Man-Made Breast.* New Brunswick, NJ: Rutgers University Press.

Jaffe, Paul. 1995. "History and Overview of Adulthood ADD." Pp. 3–17 in Kathleen G. Nadeau (ed.), *A Comprehensive Guide to Attention Deficit Disorder in Adults: Research, Diagnosis, and Treatment.* New York: Brunner/Mazel.

JAMA editorial. 1903. "Prophylaxis of Baldness." *Journal of the American Medical Association* 40: 249.

Janowitz, Morris. 1975. "Sociological Theory and Social Control." *American Journal of Sociology* 81: 82–108.

Jenness, Valerie. 1995. "Social Movement Growth, Domain Expansion, and Framing Process: The Gay/Lesbian Movement and Violence against Gays and Lesbians as a Social Problem." *Social Problems* 43: 145–63.

Joffe, Carole. 1982. "Review of Deviance and Medicalization: From Badness to Sickness." *Social Science and Medicine* 16: 921.

Johnson, Carla K. 2006. "Hormone Offers Promise of Youth, Risks." Associated Press, March 19.

Johnson, Dale L. 1998. "Are Mental Health Services Losing Out in the U.S. under Managed Care?" *PharmacoEconomics* 14 (6): 597–601.

Juengst, Eric T. 1998. "What Does Enhancement Mean?" In Erik Parens (ed.), *Enhancing Human Traits: Ethical and Social Implications.* Washington, D.C.: Georgetown University Press.

Jureidini, John N., Christopher J. Doecke, Peter R. Mansfield, et al. 2004. "Efficacy and Safety of Antidepressants for Children and Adolescents." *British Medical Journal* 328: 879–83.

Kadison, Richard. 2005. "Getting an Edge: Use of Stimulants and Antidepressants in College." *New England Journal of Medicine* 353: 1089–91.

Kaiser Family Foundation. 2005. "Non-Federal Physicians per 100,000 Civilian Population, 1970–2003" (Exhibit 5–7). *Trends and Indicators in the Changing Health Care Marketplace.* www.kff.org/insurance/7031/ti20045-7.cfm.

Kallmann, Franz J. 1952. "Comparative Twin Studies on the Genetic Aspects of Male Homosexuality." *Journal of Nervous and Mental Disease* 115: 283–98.

Kass, Leon, et al. 2003. "Medicalization: Its Nature, Causes, and Consequences." Transcript of June 12 session of the President's Council on Bioethics. www.bioethics.gov/transcripts/jun03/session2.html.

Katz, Stephen, and Barbara Marshall. 2004. "New Sex for Old: Lifestyle, Consumerism, and the Ethics of Aging Well." *Journal of Aging Studies* 17: 3–16.

Kaufman, M. 2003. "FDA Approves Wider Use of Growth Hormone." *Washington Post,* July 26, A12.

Kaufman, Sharon R., Janet K. Shim, and Ann J. Russ. 2004. "Revisiting the Biomedicalization of Aging: Clinical Trends and Ethical Changes." *Gerontologist* 44: 731–38.

Kaw, Eugenia. 1992. "Medicalization of Racial Features: Asian American Women and Cosmetic Surgery." *Medical Anthropology Quarterly* 7: 74–87.

Kawachi, Ichiro, and Peter Conrad. 1996. "Medicalization and the Pharmacological Treatment of Blood Pressure." Pp. 26–41 in P. Davis (ed.), *Contested Ground: Public Purpose and Private Interest in the Regulation of Prescription Drugs.* New York: Oxford University Press.

Kayal, Philip. 1993. *Bearing Witness: Gay Men's Health Crisis and the Politics of AIDS.* Boulder, CO: Westview.

Kearns, Walter. 1939. "The Clinical Application of Testosterone." *Journal of the American Medical Association* 112: 2257.

Keating, Nancy L., Paul D. Cleary, Alice S. Rossi, et al. 1999. "Use of Hormone Replacement Therapy by Postmenopausal Women in the United States." *Annals of Internal Medicine* 130 (7): 545–53.

Kelleher, Susan, and Duff Wilson. 2005. "Suddenly Sick: The Hidden Big Business behind Your Doctor's Diagnosis." *Seattle Times.* Special reprint of a series published June 26–30.

Kelly, Kate, and Peggy Ramundo. 1993. *You Mean I'm Not Lazy, Stupid, or Crazy?! A Self-Help Book for Adults with Attention Deficit Disorder.* Cincinnati: Tyrell and Jerem.

Kelnar, C. J. H., K. Albertsson-Wikland, R. L. Hintz, et al. 1999. "Should We Treat Children with Idiopathic Short Stature?" *Hormone Research* 52: 150–57.

Kenan, Regina H. 1996. "The At-Risk Health Status and Technology: A Diagnostic Invitation and the 'Gift' of Knowing." *Social Science and Medicine* 42: 1545–53.

Kessler, Ronald C., Patricia Berglund, Olga Demler, et al. 2005a. "Lifetime Prevalence and Age-of-Onset Distributions of DSM-IV Disorders in the National Comorbidity Survey Replication." *Archives of General Psychiatry* 62: 593–602.

Kessler, Ronald C., W. T. Chiu, O. Demler, and E. E. Walters. 2005b. "Prevalence, Severity, and Co-Morbidity of 12 Month DSM-IV Disorders in the National Co-Morbidity Replication (NCS-R)." *Archives of General Psychiatry* 62: 629–40.

Kessler, Ronald C., Olga Demler, Richard G. Frank, et al. 2005c. "Prevalence and Treatment of Mental Disorders, 1990–2003." *New England Journal of Medicine* 352: 2515–23.

Kessler, Ronald C., L. Adler, R. Barkley, et al. 2006a. "The Prevalence and Correlates of Adult ADHD in the United States: Results from the National Comorbidity Survey Replication." *American Journal of Psychiatry* 163: 716–23.

Kessler, Ronald C., E. F. Coccaro, L. M. Fava, et al. 2006b. "The Prevalence and Correlates of DSM-IV Intermittent Explosive Disorder in the National Comorbidity Replication." *Archives of General Psychiatry* 63: 669–78.

Keyes, Robert. 1980. *The Height of Your Life*. Boston: Little, Brown.

Khan, Sajjad, and Dow B. Stough. 1996. "Determination of Hairline Placement." Pp. 425–29 in Dow B. Stough and Robert S. Haber (eds.), *Hair Replacement: Surgical and Medical*. St. Louis: Mosby.

Kicman, Andrew T., and David A. Cowan. 1992. "Peptide Hormones and Sport: Misuse and Detection." *British Medical Bulletin* 48: 496–517.

Kirk, Stuart A. 2005. "Are We All Going Mad, or Are the Experts Crazy?" *Los Angeles Times*, August 14, M5.

Kirk, Stuart, and Herb Kutchins. 1992. *The Selling of DSM: The Rhetoric of Science in Psychiatry*. New York: Aldine de Gruyter.

Klawiter, Maren. 1998. "Risk, Prevention, and the Breast Cancer Continuum: The NCI, the FDA, Health Activism, and the Pharmaceutical Industry." *History and Technology* 18: 309–53.

Klerman, Gerald. 1972. "Psychotropic Hedonism vs. Pharmacological Calvinism." *Hastings Center Report* 2 (4): 1–3.

Koerner, Brendan I. 2002. "Disorders, Made to Order." *Mother Jones* 27: 58–63.

Kolata, Gina. 1996. "Boom in Ritalin Sales Raises Ethical Issues." *New York Times*, May 15, C8.

———. 2003. "Panel Recommends Studies on Testosterone Therapy." *New York Times*, November 13, A22.

———. 2005. "Rapid Rise and Fall for Body-Scanning Clinics." *New York Times*, January 23, 1.

Konner, Melvin J. 1999. "One Pill Makes You Larger: The Ethics of Enhancement." *American Prospect* 42: 55–60.

Krajeski, James. 1996. "Homosexuality and the Mental Health Profession." Pp. 17–31 in Robert Cabaj and Terry Stein (eds.), *Textbook of Homosexuality and Mental Health*. Washington, D.C.: American Psychiatric Press.

Kramer, Peter. 1993. *Listening to Prozac*. New York: Penguin Books.

Kroll-Smith, Steve. 2003. "Popular Media and 'Excessive Daytime Sleepiness': A Study of Rhetorical Authority in Medical Sociology." In Clive Seale (ed.), *Health in the Media (Sociology of Health and Illness Monograph Series)*. Oxford: Blackwell.

Kroll-Smith, Steve, Phil Brown, and Valerie Gunter. 2000. *Illness in the Environment: A Reader in Contested Medicine*. New York: New York University Press.

Kroll-Smith, Steve, and H. Hugh Floyd. 1997. *Bodies in Protest: Environmental Illness and the Struggle over Medical Knowledge*. New York: New York University Press.

Kutchins, Herb, and Stuart A. Kirk. 1997. *Making Us Crazy: DSM: The Psychiatric Bible and the Creation of Mental Disorders*. New York: New York University Press.

Lantos, J., M. Siegler, and L. Cutler. 1989. "Ethical Issues in Growth Hormone Therapy." *Journal of the American Medical Association* 261: 1020–24.

Lakoff, Andrew. 2005. *Pharmaceutical Reason: Knowledge and Value in Global Psychiatry*. New York: Cambridge University Press.

Latham, Patricia H., and Peter S. Latham. 1992. *Attention Deficit Disorder and the Law: A Guide for Advocates*. Washington, D.C.: JKL Communications.

Latham, Peter S., and Patricia H. Latham. 1995. "Legal Rights of the ADD Adult." Pp. 337–50 in Kathleen G. Nadeau (ed.), *A Comprehensive Guide to Attention Deficit Disorder in Adults*. New York: Brunner/Mazel.

Laumann, Edward O., Anthony Paik, and Raymond C. Rosen. 1999. "Sexual Dysfunction in the United States." *Journal of the American Medical Association* 281:537–44.

Lee, Ellie. 2003. *Abortion, Motherhood, and Mental Health: Medicalizing Reproduction in the United States and Great Britain*. New York: Aldine de Gruyter.

Leffers, Jeanne Mahoney. 1997. "The Social Construction of a New Diagnostic Category: Attention Deficit Disorder in Adults (Medicalization)." Ph.D. diss., Brown University.

Lenzer, Jeanne. 2005. "American Medical Association Rejects Proposal to Ban Consumer Adverts for Prescription Medicines." *British Medical Journal* 331: 7.

LeVay, Simon. 1991. "A Difference in the Hypothalmic Structure between Heterosexual and Homosexual Men." *Science* 253: 1034–37.

LeVay, Simon, and Dean Hamer. 1994. "Evidence for a Biological Influence in Male Homosexuality." *Scientific American* 270 (5): 44–49.

Light, Donald W. 1993. "Countervailing Power: The Changing Character of the Medical Profession in the United States." Pp. 69–80 in F. W. Hafferty and J. B. McKinlay (eds.), *The Changing Medical Profession: An International Perspective*. New York: Oxford University Press.

Lindenman, B. 1993. "Danger in the Fountain of Youth." *Record*, December 9, B04.

Livingston, Ken. 1997. "Ritalin: Miracle Drug or Cop-Out?" *Public Interest* 127 (spring): 3–18.

Lock, Margaret. 1993. *Encounters with Aging: Mythologies of Menopause in Japan and North America*. Berkeley: University of California Press.

———. 2001. "Medicalization: Cultural Concerns." Pp. 9534–39 in Neil J. Smelser and Paul B. Baltes (eds.), *International Encyclopedia of the Social and Behavioral Sciences*. New York: Elsevier.

———. 2004. "Medicalization and the Naturalization of Social Control." Pp. 116–24 in Carol R. Ember and Melvin Ember (eds.), *Encyclopedia of Medical Anthropology*, vol. 1. New York: Springer.

Loe, Meika. 2001. "Fixing Broken Masculinity: Viagra Technology for the Production of Gender and Sexuality." *Sexuality and Culture* 5: 97–125.

———. 2004. *The Rise of Viagra: How the Little Blue Pill Changed Sex in America*. New York: New York University Press.

Loseke, Donileen R. 1999. *Thinking about Social Problems*. New York: Aldine de Gruyter.

Lowenberg, June S., and Fred Davis. 1994. "Beyond Medicalization-Demedicalization: The Case of Holistic Health." *Sociology of Health and Illness* 16: 579–99.

Luciano, Lynne. 2001. *Looking Good: Male Body Image in Modern America.* New York: Hill and Wang.

Lupton, Deborah. 1993. "Risk as Moral Danger: The Social and Political Functions of Risk Discourse in Public Health." *International Journal of Health Services* 23: 425–35.

———. 1997. "Foucault and the Medicalization Critique." Pp. 94–112 in Alan Peterson and Robin Bunton (eds.), *Foucault: Health and Medicine.* London: Routledge.

Mahler, Jonathan. 2004. "The Antidepressant Dilemma." *New York Times Magazine,* November 21.

Majumdar, Sumit R., Elizabeth A. Almasi, and Randall S. Stafford. 2004. "Promotion and Prescribing of Hormone Replacement Therapy after Report of Harm by the Women's Health Initiative." *Journal of the American Medical Association* 292 (16): 1983–88.

Malacrida, Claudia. 2003. *Cold Comfort: Mothers, Professionals, and Attention Deficit Disorder.* Toronto: University of Toronto Press.

Mamo, Laura, and Jennifer Fishman. 2001. "Potency in All the Right Places: Viagra as a Gendered Technology of the Body." *Body and Society* 7 (4): 13–35.

Mannuzza, Salvatore, Rachel Gittleman Klein, and Kathy A. Addalli. 1991. "Young Adult Mental Status of Hyperactive Boys and Their Brothers: A Prospective Follow-up Study." *Journal of the American Academy of Child and Adolescent Psychiatry* 30 (5): 743–51.

Mannuzza, Salvatore, Rachel G. Klein, Abrah Bressler, et al. 1998. "Adult Psychiatric Status of Hyperactive Boys Grown Up." *American Journal of Psychiatry* 155 (4): 493–98.

Marino, Vivian. 2002. "All Those Commercials Pay off for Drug Makers." *New York Times,* February 24, sec. 3, p. 4.

Marritt, Emanuel. 1996. "The Overwhelming Responsibility." Pp. 299–312 in Dow B. Stough and Robert S. Haber (eds.), *Hair Replacement: Surgical and Medical.* St. Louis: Mosby.

Marritt, Emanuel, and Leonard M. Dzubow. 1996. "Reassessment of Male Pattern Baldness: A Reevaluation of the Treatment." Pp. 30–41 in Dow B. Stough and Robert S. Haber (eds.), *Hair Replacement: Surgical and Medical.* St. Louis: Mosby.

Marshall, Barbara L., and Stephen Katz. 2002. "Forever Functional: Sexual Fitness and the Ageing Male Body." *Body and Society* 8: 43–70.

Marshall, Eliot. 2004. "Antidepressants and Children: Buried Data Can Be Hazardous to a Company's Health." *Science* 304: 1576–77.

Martel, Leslie F., and Henry B. Biller. 1987. *Stature and Stigma: The Biopsychological Development of Short Males.* Lexington, MA: Lexington Books.

Martin, Emily. 1987. *The Woman in the Body: A Cultural Analysis of Reproduction.* Boston: Beacon.

Mathews, Jay. 1999. "The Shrinking Field." *Washington Post,* August 2, C01.

May, Carl. 2001. "Pathology, Identity, and the Social Construction of Alcohol Dependence." *Sociology* 35: 385–401.

Mayes, Rick, and Allan V. Horwitz. 2005. "DSM-III and the Revolution in the Classification of Mental Illness." *Journal of the History of Behavioral Sciences* 41: 249–68.

McCrea, Frances B. 1983. "The Politics of Menopause: The 'Discovery' of a Deficiency Disease." *Social Problems* 31: 111–23.

McDowell, Jim. 1997. "A Hyperactive Way to Make More Money: Teens with Ritalin Prescriptions Can Supply Drug-Abusing Classmates." *British Columbia Report* 8 (28): 34–35.

McKinlay, John B., and A. Gemmel. 2003. "Hormone Replacement Therapy/Policy." Unpublished manuscript, New England Research Institute, Watertown, MA.

McKinlay, John B., and Lisa D. Marceau. 2002. "The End of the Golden Age of Doctoring." *International Journal of Health Services* 32 (2): 379–416.

McLaughlin, Lisa, and Alice Park. 2000. "Are You Man Enough?" *Time*, April 24, 58–63.

McLeod, Jane D., Bernice A. Pescosolido, David T. Takeuchi, and Terry Falkenberg White. 2004. "Public Attitudes toward the Use of Psychiatric Medications for Children." *Journal of Health and Social Behavior* 45: 53–67.

Meador, Clifton. 1994. "The Last Well Person." *New England Journal of Medicine* 330: 440–41.

Mehlman, Maxwell J. 2000. "The Law of Above Averages: Leveling the New Genetic Enhancement Playing Field." *Iowa Law Review* 85: 517–93.

Meyer, Alfred. 1996. "Listening to Paxil." *Psychology Today*, July/August, 60–70.

Mintz, Howard. 1995. "A Growing Problem: The Minnesota Acquittal of a Genentech Official Spells Problems for S.F. Prosecutors." *Recorder*, November 8, 1.

Morley, J. E., and H. M. Perry III. 2003. "Androgen Treatment of Male Hypogonadism in Older Males." *Journal of Steroid Biochemistry and Molecular Biology* 85: 367–73.

Morris, Rebecca, Liu Yaping, Marles Lee, et al. 2004. "Capturing and Profiling Hair Follicle Stem Cells." *Nature Biotechnology* 22: 411–17.

Moynihan, Ray. 2003. "The Making of a Disease: Female Sexual Dysfunction." *British Medical Journal* 326: 45–47.

Moynihan, Ray, and Alan Cassels. 2005. *Selling Sickness: How the World's Biggest Pharmaceutical Companies Are Turning Us All into Patients.* New York: Nation Books.

Muiderman, Kevin. 2001. "Hair Restoration Surgery through Micrografting Techniques." *Plastic Surgical Nursing* 21: 141–42.

Mumford, Kevin. 1992. "Lost Manhood Found: Male Sexual Impotence and Victorian Culture in the United States." *Journal of the History of Sexuality* 3: 33–77.

Murray, M. D., and F. W. Deardorff. 1998. "Does Managed Care Fuel Pharmaceutical Industry Growth?" *PharmacoEconomics* 14 (4): 341–48.

Murray, Stephen. 1996. *American Gay.* Chicago: University of Chicago Press.

Mykytyn, Courtney Everts. 2006. "Anti-Aging Medicine: A Patient/Practitioner Movement to Redefine Aging." *Social Science and Medicine* 62: 643–53.

Nadeau, Kathleen G. (ed.) 1995a. *A Comprehensive Guide to Attention Deficit Disorder in Adults: Research, Diagnosis, and Treatment.* New York: Brunner/Mazel.

——. 1995b. "ADD in the Workplace: Career Consultation and Counseling for the Adult with ADD." In Kathleen G. Nadeau (ed.), *A Comprehensive Guide to Attention Deficit Disorder in Adults: Research, Diagnosis, and Treatment.* New York: Brunner/Mazel.

Navarro, Vicente. 1976. *Medicine under Capitalism.* New York: Prodist.

Newcorn, Jeffrey H., Jeffrey M. Halperin, James M. Healey, et al. 1989. "Are ADDH and ADHD the Same or Different?" *Journal of the American Academy of Adolescent Psychiatry* 285: 734–38.

New York Times. 1990. "Not Quite the Fountain of Youth." July 6, A24.

——. 1996. "Growth Hormone Fails to Reverse Effects of Aging, Researchers Say." April 15, A13.

——. 1999. "For School Nurses, More Than Tending the Sick." January 18.

——. 2006. "Industry's Role in Hypertension." Editorial. May 30. http://www.google.com /search?hl=en&lr=&client=safari&rls=en&q=Hypertension+Times++ May +30&btnG=Search.

Newsweek. 1985. "A Hormone with Growth Potential." November 25, 70.

————. 1990. "A New View on Hyperactivity." December 3, 61.

NHANES (National Health and Nutrition Examination Survey). 2000. *2000 CDC Growth Charts: United States.* Washington, D.C.: National Center for Health Statistics. www.cdc.gov/growth charts.

Nieschlag, E., and H. M. Behre (eds.). 1998. *Testosterone: Action, Deficiency, and Substitution.* New York: Springer.

NIHCM (National Institute for Health Care Management). 2001. *Prescription Drug Expenditures in 2000: The Upward Trend Continues.* Washington, D.C.: NIHCM.

Nissen, Steven F. 2006. "ADHD Drugs and Cardiovascular Risk." *New England Journal of Medicine* 354: 1445–48.

Nordenberg, T. 1999. "Maker of Growth Hormone Feels Long Arm of Law." *FDA Consumer,* September/October, 33.

North American Menopause Society. 2003. "Position Statement: Estrogen and Progestogen Use in Peri- and Postmenopausal Women: September 2003 Position Statement of the North American Menopause Society." *Menopause: The Journal of the North American Menopause Society* 10 (6): 497–506.

Nuffield Council on Bioethics. 2002. *Genetics and Human Behaviour: The Ethical Context.* London: Nuffield Council on Bioethics.

Okie, Susan. 2006. "ADHD in Adults." *New England Journal of Medicine* 354: 2637–41.

Olfson, Mark, S. C. Marcus, M. M. Weissman, and P. S. Jensen. 2002. "National Trends in the Use of Psychotropic Medications by Children." *Journal of the American Academy of Child and Adolescent Psychiatry* 41: 514–21.

Olfson, Mark, Marc J. Gameroff, Steven C. Marcus, and Peter S. Jensen. 2003. "National Trends in the Treatment of Attention Deficit Hyperactivity Disorder." *American Journal of Psychiatry* 160: 1071–77.

Oliver, Mike. 1996. *Understanding Disability: From Theory to Practice.* Basingstoke, UK: Macmillan.

Papadakis, Maxine A., Deborah Grady, Dennis Black, et al. 1996. "Growth Hormone Replacement in Healthy Older Men Improves Body Composition but Not Functional Ability." *Annals of Internal Medicine* 124: 8–16.

Parens, Erik. 1998. "Is Better Always Good? The Enhancement Project." In Erik Parens (ed.), *Enhancing Human Traits: Ethical and Social Implications.* Washington, D.C.: Georgetown University Press.

Parker, W. 1994. Testimony before the House Committee on Business, Subcommittee on Regulation, Business Opportunities, and Technology, on the Questionable Practices in Drug Industry Marketing and Promotion, 12 October, 106th Cong., 1st sess.

Parsons, Talcott. 1951. *The Social System.* Glencoe: Free Press.

Patlak, Margie. 1992. "The Long and Short of It: New Medications for Growth Disorders." *FDA Consumer* 26: 30–35.

Paul, Diane. 1995. *Controlling Human Heredity: 1865 to the Present.* Atlantic Highlands, NJ: Humanities.

Pawluch, Dorothy. 1983. "Transitions in Pediatrics: A Segmental Analysis." *Social Problems* 30: 449–65.

PBS (Public Broadcasting Service). 1995. "ADD: A Dubious Diagnosis." *Merrow Report,* October 20.

Pear, Robert. 2006. "Growth of National Health Spending Slows along with Drug Sales." *New York Times,* 20 January, A15.

Perls, Thomas T., Neal R. Reisman, and Jay Olshansky. 2005. "Provision or Distribution of Growth Hormone for 'Antiaging': Clinical and Legal Issues." *Journal of the American Medical Association* 294: 1993.

Petersen, Alan R. 1998. *Unmasking the Masculine: 'Men' and 'Identity' in a Sceptical Age*. London: Sage.

Peterson, Melody. 2002. "Advertising: Judge Orders Drug Company to Alter Ads." *New York Times*, August 21, C1.

Pillard, Richard C., and J. D. Weinrich. 1986. "Evidence of Familial Nature of Male Homosexuality." *Archives of General Psychiatry* 43: 808–12.

Pitts, Jesse. 1968. "Social Control: The Concept." *International Encyclopedia of Social Sciences* 14. New York: Macmillan.

Pleak, Richard. 1999. "Ethical Issues in Diagnosing and Treating Gender-Dysphoric Children and Adolescents." Pp. 34–51 in Matthew Rottneck (ed.), *Sissies and Tomboys: Gender Nonconformity and Homosexual Childhood*. New York: New York University Press.

PLoS Medicine. 2006. *Public Library of Science* 3 (4). plosmedicine.org.

Pollack, Andrew. 2005. "Marketing a Disease, and Also a Drug to Treat It." *New York Times*, May 9, 1.

Press, Nancy. 2006. "Social Construction and Medicalization: Behavioral Genetics in Context." Pp. 131–49 in Erik Perens, Audrey R. Chapman, and Nancy Press (eds.), *Wrestling with Behavioral Genetics: Science, Ethics, and Public Conversation*. Baltimore: Johns Hopkins University Press.

Price, F. 1994. Statement prepared for the House Committee on Business, Subcommittee on Regulation, Business Opportunities, and Technology, on the Questionable Practices in Drug Industry Marketing and Promotion, 12 October, 106th Cong., 1st sess.

Public Citizen. 2003. "2002 Drug Industry Profits: Hefty Pharmaceutical Company Margins Dwarf Other Industries." Retrieved July 15, 2004. www.citizen.org/documents/Pharma_Report.pdf.

Quinn, Brian. 2001. "The Medicalisation of Online Behavior." *Online Information Review* 25: 173–80.

Rae, S. 1996. "Hormones: Natural Age-Erasers." *Men's Health* 11: 65–66.

Rafalovich, Adam. 2004. *Framing ADHD Children: A Critical Examination of the History, Discourse, and Everyday Experience of Attention Deficit/Hyperactivity Disorder*. Lanham, MD: Lexington Books.

Ramos e Silva, Marcia. 2000. "Male Pattern Hair Loss: Prevention Rather Than Regrowth." *International Journal of Dermatology* 39: 728–31.

Randall, Valerie A. 2000. "The Biology of Androgenetic Alopecia." Pp. 123–33 in Francisco Camacho, Valerie Randall, and Vera Price (eds.), *Hair and Its Disorders: Biology, Pathology, and Management*. London: Martin Dunitz.

Ratey, John J., Mark S. Greenberg, Jules R. Bemporad, and Karen J. Lindem. 1992. "Unrecognized Attention-Deficit Hyperactivity Disorder in Adults Presenting for Outpatient Psychotherapy." *Journal of Child and Adolescent Psychopharmacology* 2: 267–75.

Relman, Arnold S., and Marcia Angell, 2002. "America's Other Drug Problem." *New Republic*, December 16, 27–41.

Rice, G., C. Anderson, N. Reich, and G. Ebers. 1999. "Male Homosexuality: Absence of Linkage to Microsatellite Markers at Xq28." *Science* 284: 665–67.

Rich, Adrienne, 1980. "Compulsory Heterosexuality and Lesbian Experience." *Signs: Journal of Women in Culture and Society* 5: 631–60.

Riessman, Catherine Kohler. 1983. "Women and Medicalization: A New Perspective." *Social Policy* 14 (summer): 3–18.

Riska, Elianne. 2003. "Gendering the Medicalization Thesis." *Advances in Gender Research* 7: 61–89.

Rosack, Jim. 2005. "New Data Shows Declines in Antidepressant Prescribing." *Psychiatric News* 40 (7): 1.

Rose, Steven. 2005. *The Future of the Brain: The Promise and Perils of Tomorrow's Neuroscience.* New York: Oxford University Press.

Rosenberg, Charles. 2000. "Banishing Risk: Continuity and Change in Moral Management of Disease." In A. Brandt and P. Rozin (eds.), *Morality and Health.* New York: Routledge.

Rosenfeld, Dana, and Christopher A. Faircloth (eds.). 2006. *Medicalized Masculinities.* Philadelphia: Temple University Press.

Rosenthal, Meredith B., Ernst R. Berndt, Julie M. Donohue, et al. 2002. "Promotion of Prescription Drugs to Consumers." *New England Journal of Medicine* 346: 498–505.

Rossol, Josh. 2001. "The Medicalization of Deviance as an Interactive Achievement: The Construction of Compulsive Gambling." *Symbolic Interaction* 24: 315–41.

Rothman, David J. 2001. "Comments on Genetic Enhancement." Talk given at plenary session of tenth-anniversary ELSI (Ethical, Legal, and Social Implications of the Human Genome Project) conference, 17 January, Washington, D.C.

Rothman, Sheila M., and David J. Rothman. 2003. *The Pursuit of Perfection: The Promise and Perils of Medical Enhancement.* New York: Pantheon Books.

Rubin, Henry S. 2003. *Self-Made Men.* Nashville: Vanderbilt University Press.

Rubin, Rita. 2005. "C-Section Rate Hits Record High at 29%." *USA Today,* 16 November, D9.

——. 2006. "Warnings Advised on ADHD Drugs: FDA Committee Urges Strongest Notification." *USA Today,* February 10.

Rudman, Daniel, A. G. Feller, G. A. Nagraj, et al. 1990. "Effects of Human Growth Hormone in Men over 60 Years Old." *New England Journal of Medicine* 323: 1–6.

Rudman, Daniel, A. G. Feller, L. Cohn, et al. 1991. "Effects of Human Growth Hormone on Body Composition in Elderly Men." *Hormone Research* 36, suppl. 1: 73–81.

Sadie, Stanley (ed.) and John Tyrrell (exec. ed.). 2001. *The New Grove Dictionary of Music and Musicians,* 2nd ed. London: Macmillan

Salant, Talya, and Heena P. Santry. 2006. "Internet Marketing of Bariatric Surgery: Contemporary Trends in the Medicalization of Obesity." *Social Science and Medicine* 62: 2445–57.

Sallah, Anna. 2004. "Doping Tests May Fail in Court." www.abc.au/science/news/stories/s1164674.htim. Accessed in 2004.

Saltus, Richard. 1990. "Tinkering with the Mechanisms of Aging." *Boston Globe,* August 6, 25.

——. 1996. "Youth in a Bottle?" *Boston Globe,* December 8, 12.

Samaras, Thomas T. 1995. "Short Is Beautiful: So Why Are We Making Kids Grow Tall?" *Futurist* 29: 26–30.

Sandberg, David E. 1999. "Experiences of Being Short: Should We Expect Problems in Psychosocial Adjustment." Pp. 15–26 in U. Eiholzer, F. Haverkamp, and L. Voss (eds.), *Growth, Stature, and Psychosocial Well-Being.* Seattle: Hogrefe and Huber.

Saugy, M. C., C. Cardis, C. Schweizer, et al. 1996. "Detection of Human Growth Hormone in Urine: Out of Competition Tests Are Necessary." *Journal of Chromatography* B587: 201–11.

Saul, Stephanie. 2006. "Unease on Industry's Role in Hypertension Debate." *New York Times,* May 20, 1.

Sault, Nicole (ed.). 1994. *Many Mirrors: Body Image and Social Relations.* New Brunswick, NJ: Rutgers University Press.

Savin-Williams, Ritch. 2001. "Memories of Same-Sex Attractions." Pp. 117–33 in Michael Kimmel and Michael Messner (eds.), *Men's Lives*. Boston: Allyn and Bacon.

Scheff, Thomas J. 1984. *Being Mentally Ill: A Sociological Theory*, rev. ed. Chicago: Aldine.

Scheper-Hughes, Nancy, and Margaret M. Lock. 1987. "The Mindful Body: A Prolegomenon to Future Work in Medical Anthropology." *Medical Anthropology Quarterly* 1: 6–41.

Schneider, Joseph W. 1978. "Deviant Drinking as a Disease: Alcoholism as a Social Accomplishment." *Social Problems* 25: 361–72.

Schrag, Peter, and Diane Divoky. 1976. *Myth of the Hyperactive Child*. New York: Pantheon.

Schulz, Kathryn. 2004. "Did Antidepressants Depress Japan?" *New York Times Magazine*, August 22, 38–41,

Schumacher, A. 1982. "On the Significance of Short Stature in Human Society." *Journal of Human Evolution* 11: 697–701.

Schur, Edwin. 1976. *The Awareness Trap: Self Absorption Instead of Social Change*. New York: Quadrangle/New York Times Books.

Schwartz, Hillel. 1986. *Never Satisfied: A Cultural History of Diet, Fantasies, and Fat*. New York: Free Press.

Schwartz, Lisa M., and Steven Woloshin. 2003. "On the Prevention and Treatment of Exaggeration." *Journal of General Internal Medicine* 18 (2): 153–54.

Science News. 1999. "Gene Therapy Tackles Hair Loss." October 30, 283.

Scott, Susie. 2006. "The Medicalisation of Shyness: From Social Misfits to Social Fitness." *Sociology of Health and Illness* 28: 133–53.

Scott, Wilbur J. 1990. "PTSD in DSM-III: A Case of the Politics of Diagnosis and Disease." *Social Problems* 37: 294–310.

Scow, Dean Thomas, Robert S. Nolte, and Allen F. Shaughnessy. 1999. "Medical Treatments for Balding in Men." *American Family Physician*, April 15.

Searight, H. Russell, and A. Lesley McLaren. 1998. "Attention-Deficit Hyperactivity Disorder: The Medicalization of Misbehavior." *Journal of Clinical Psychology in Medical Settings* 5 (4): 467–95.

Segal, Judy Z. 2005. *Health and the Rhetoric of Medicine*. Carbondale: Southern Illinois University Press.

Segrave, Kerry. 1996. *Baldness: A Social History*. Jefferson, NC: McFarland.

Seidman, Steven. 2001. "From Identity to Queer Politics: Shifts in Normative Heterosexuality and the Meaning of Citizenship." *Citizenship Studies* 5 (3): 321–28.

Shaffer, David. 1994. "Attention Deficit Hyperactivity Disorder in Adults." *American Journal of Psychiatry* 151: 633–38.

Shapiro, Joseph. 1994. "Disability Policy and the Media: A Stealth Civil Rights Movement Bypasses the Press and Defies Conventional Wisdom." *Policy Studies Journal* 22: 123–32.

Shaw, Ian, and Louise Woodward. 2004. "The Medicalization of Unhappiness? The Management of Mental Distress in Primary Care." In Ian Shaw and Kaisa Kauppinen (eds.), *Constructions of Health and Illness: European Perspectives*. Aldershot, UK: Ashgate.

Shell-Duncan, Bettina. 2001. "The Medicalization of Female 'Circumcision': Harm Reduction or Promotion of a Dangerous Practice?" *Social Science and Medicine* 52: 1013–28.

Shilts, Randy. 1987. *And the Band Played On: Politics, People, and the AIDS Epidemic*. New York: St. Martin's.

Shore, Miles F., and A. Beigel. 1996. "The Challenges Posed by Managed Behavioral Health Care." *New England Journal of Medicine* 334: 116–18.

Shumaker, Sally A., Claudine Legault, Stephen R. Rapp, et al., for the WHIMS investigators. 2002. "Estrogen Plus Progestin and the Incidence of Dementia and Mild Cognitive Impairment in Postmenopausal Women: The Women's Health Initiative Memory Study: A Randomized Controlled Trial," *Journal of the American Medical Association* 289: 2651–62.

Silver, Lee M. 1997. *Remaking Eden: Cloning and Beyond in a Brave New World.* New York: Avon Books.

Silverstein, Ken. 1999. "Prozac.org." *Mother Jones,* November–December. http://www.motherjones.com/news/feature/1999/11/nami.html.

Sinclair, Rodney. 1998. "Male Pattern Androgenetic Alopecia." *British Journal of Medicine* 317: 865–69.

Singer, Merrill, Carol Arnold, Maureen Fitzgerald, et al. 1984. "Hypoglycemia: A Controversial Illness in U.S. Society." *Medical Anthropology* 8: 1–35.

Slater, Lauren. 2001. "Dr. Daedalus." *Harper's Magazine,* July, 57–67.

Smith, Richard. 2005. "Medical Journals Are an Extension of the Marketing Arm of Pharmaceutical Companies." *PLoS Medicine* 2 (5): 346–66.

Smith, Stephen. 2003. "Hormone Therapy's Rise and Fall: Science Lost Its Way and Women Lost Out." *Boston Globe,* July 20, A1.

Sobal, Jeffery, and Donna Maurer (eds.). 1995. *Eating Agendas: Food and Nutrition as Social Problems.* New York: Aldine de Gruyter.

Sontag, Susan. 1978. *Illness as Metaphor.* New York: Farrar, Straus, and Giroux.

Stabinger, K. 1999. "Potent Mix: Taxing Hormones and Supplements to Combat Aging." *Vogue,* January, 162–63.

Stallings, Robert A. 1990. "Media Discourse and the Social Construction of Risk." *Social Problems* 37: 80–95.

Stapleton, S. 1999. "More Off Label Drug Promotion in the Offing." *American Medical News,* August, 25–30.

Starr, Paul. 1982. *The Social Transformation of American Medicine.* New York: Basic Books.

Stas, Sameer N., Aristotelis G. Anastasiadis, Harry Fisch, et al. 2003. "Urologic Aspects of Andropause." *Urology* 61: 261–66.

Stein, Edward. 1999. *The Mismeasure of Desire: The Science, Theory, and Ethics of Sexual Orientation.* New York: Oxford University Press.

Stephenson, J. 2003. "FDA Orders Estrogen Safety Warnings: Agency Offers Guidance for HRT Use." *Journal of the American Medical Association* 289: 537–38.

Stevens, Patricia E., and Joanne M. Hall. 1991. "A Critical Historical Analysis of the Medical Construction of Lesbianism." *International Journal of Health Services* 21: 291–308.

Stewart, Mark A. 1970. "Hyperactive Children." *Scientific American* 222: 794–98.

Stewart, Mark A., A. Ferris, N. P. Pitts, and A. G. Craig. 1966. "The Hyperactive Child Syndrome." *American Journal of Orthopsychiatry* 36: 861–67.

Stich, Sally. 1993. "Why Can't Your Husband Sit Still?" *Ladies' Home Journal,* September, 74–77.

Stoudemire, Alan. 1996. "Psychiatry in Medical Practice: Implications for the Education of Primary Care Physicians in the Era of Managed Care. Part 1." *Psychosomatics* 37: 502–8.

Stough, Dow B., and Robert S. Haber (eds). 1996. *Hair Replacement: Surgical and Medical.* St. Louis: Mosby.

Strong, Phil. 1979. "Sociological Imperialism and the Profession of Medicine: A Critical Examination of the Thesis of Medical Imperialism." *Social Science and Medicine* 13A: 199–215.

Sullivan, Deborah A. 2001. *Cosmetic Surgery: The Cutting Edge of Medicine in America.* New Brunswick, NJ: Rutgers University Press.

Sultan, Faye, Denise Elsner, and Jaime Smith. 1987. "Ego-Dystonic Homosexuality and Treatment Alternatives." Pp. 187–97 in Louis Diamont (ed.), *Male and Female Homosexuality: Psychological Approaches.* New York: Hemisphere.

Swidey, Neal. 2005. "What Makes People Gay?" *Boston Globe Magazine,* August 14.

Szasz, Thomas. 1970. *Manufacture of Madness.* New York: Dell.

Szymczak, Julia E., and Peter Conrad. 2006. "Medicalizing the Aging Male Body: Andropause and Baldness." In Dana Rosenfeld and Christopher Faircloth (eds.), *Medicalized Masculinities.* Philadelphia: Temple University Press.

Taaffe, D. R., L. Pruitt, J. Reim, et al. 1994. "Effect of Recombinant Human Growth Hormone on the Muscle Strength Response to Resistance Exercise in Elderly Men." *Journal of Clinical Endocrinology and Metabolism* 79: 1361–66.

Tan, Robert S., and John W. Culberson. 2003. "An Integrative Review on Current Evidence in Testosterone Replacement Therapy for the Andropause." *Maturitas* 45: 15–27.

Terry, Jennifer. 1999. *An American Obsession: Science, Medicine, and Homosexuality in Modern Society.* Chicago: University of Chicago Press.

Thomas, Cindy Parks, Peter Conrad, Rosemary Casler, and Elizabeth Goodman. 2006. "Trends in the Use of Psychotropic Medications among Adolescents, 1994–2001." *Psychiatric Services* 57: 63–69.

Thompson, Edward H. 1994. "Older Men as Invisible Men in Contemporary Society." Pp. 1–21 in Edward H. Thompson (ed.), *Older Men's Lives.* Thousand Oaks, CA: Sage.

Tiefer, Leonore. 1994. "The Medicalization of Impotence: Normalizing Phallocentricism." *Gender and Society* 8:363–77.

———. 2001a. "The 'Consensus' Conference on Female Sexual Dysfunction: Conflicts of Interest and Hidden Agendas." *Journal of Sex and Marital Therapy* 27: 227–36.

———. 2001b. "A New View of Women's Sexual Problems: Why New? Why Now?" *Journal of Sex Research* 38: 89–96.

Toby, Jackson. 1998. "Medicalizing Temptation." *Public Interest,* winter, 64–78.

Trilling, James. 1999. "My Father and the Weak-Eyed Devils." *American Scholar* 68 (2): 17–41.

Tuller, David. 2002. "Competitors to Viagra Get Ready to Rumble." *New York Times,* September 23, F7.

———. 2004. "Gentlemen, Start Your Engines." *New York Times,* June 21.

Turner, Bryan S. 1992. *Regulating Bodies: Essays in Medical Sociology.* New York: Routledge.

U.S. Department of Health and Human Services, Centers for Disease Control, National Center for Health Statistics. 2004. *Chartbook.* Washington, DC: U.S. Government Printing Office.

USA Today. 2002. "Testosterone: Shot in the Arm for Aging Males." July 26.

usolympicteam.com. 2005. "U.S. Anti-Doping Agency." www.usoc.org/12696.htm.

Van Neste, M. D. 2002. "Assessment of Hair Loss: Clinical Relevance of Hair Growth Evaluation Methods." *Clinical Dermatology* 27: 362–69.

Vance, Mary Lee. 1990. "Growth Hormone for the Elderly?" *New England Journal of Medicine* 323: 52–53.

Vastag, Brian. 2003. "Many Questions, Few Answers for Testosterone Replacement Therapy." *Journal of the American Medical Association* 289: 971–72.

Vatz, Richard E., and Lee S. Weinberg. 1997. "How Accurate Is Media Coverage of Attention Deficit Disorder?" *USA Today* 127: 76–77.

Vendantam, Shankar. 2001. "Drug Ads Hyping Anxiety Make Some Uneasy." *Washington Post*, July 16, A01.

Vincent, John A. 2006. "Ageing Contested: Anti-ageing Science and the Construction of Old Age." *Sociology* 40: 681–98.

Voss, Linda D. 1999. "Short Stature: Does It Matter? A Review of the Evidence." Pp. 7–14 in U. Eiholzer, F. Haverkamp, and L. Voss (eds.), *Growth, Stature, and Psychosocial Well-Being*. Seattle: Hogrefe and Huber.

Wagner, Jon C. 1989. "Abuse of Drugs Used to Enhance Athletic Performance." *American Journal of Hospital Pharmacy* 46: 2059–67.

Wallis, Claudia. 1994. "Life in Overdrive." *Time*, July 18, 43–50.

Warshaw, Carole. 1989. "Limitations of the Medical Model in the Care of Battered Women." *Gender and Society* 3: 506–17.

Watson, Jonathan. 2000. *Male Bodies: Health, Culture, and Identity*. Buckingham, UK: Open University Press.

Weber, Max. 1904/1958. *The Protestant Ethic and the Spirit of Capitalism*. New York: Charles Scribner's Sons.

Weintraub, Arlene. 2006. "Selling the Promise of Youth." *Business Week*, March 20, 65–74.

Weiss, Gabrielle, and Lily Trokenberg Hechtman. 1986. *Hyperactive Children Grown Up: Empirical Findings and Theoretical Considerations*. New York: Guilford.

Weiss, Gabrielle, Lily Trokenberg Hechtman, T. Perlman, et al. 1979. "Hyperactives as Young Adults: A Controlled Prospective 10-year Follow-up of the Psychiatric Status of 75 Children." *Archives of General Psychiatry* 36: 675–81.

Weiss, Lynn. 1992. *Attention Deficit Disorder in Adults: Practical Help for Sufferers and Their Spouses*. Dallas, TX. Taylor.

Weiss, Rick. 1993. "Growth Hormone Provides No Extra Inches, Study Finds Controversial Drug Does Not Add Height beyond Genetic Potential." *Washington Post*, September 13, Z7.

Wells, Pamela A., Trevor Willmouth, and Robin Russell. 1995. "Does Fortune Favor the Bald? Psychological Correlates of Hair Loss in Males." *British Journal of Psychology* 86: 337–44.

Wender, Paul H. 1971. *Minimal Brian Dysfunction in Children*. New York: Wiley.

——. 1987. *The Hyperactive Child, Adolescent, and Adult: Attention Deficit Disorder throughout the Lifespan*. New York: Oxford University Press.

——. 1995. *Attention Deficit Hyperactivity Disorder in Adults*. New York: Oxford University Press.

——. 1998. "Attention-Deficit Hyperactivity Disorder in Adults." *Psychiatry Clinic North America* 21: 761–74.

Werner, August A. 1939. "The Male Climacteric." *Journal of the American Medical Association* 112: 1441–43.

Werth, Barry. 1991. "How Short Is Too Short? Marketing Human Growth Hormone." *New York Times Magazine*, 16 June, 14–16, 28–29, 47.

Wertz, Richard, and Dorothy Wertz. 1989. *Lying In: A History of Childbirth in America*, expanded ed. New Haven: Yale University Press.

Wespes, E., and C. C. Schulman. 2002. "Male Andropause: Myth, Reality, and Treatment." *International Journal of Impotence Research* 14: S93–98.

White, Ronald D. 2002. "Judge Stays Order Halting Paxil Ads." *Los Angeles Times*, August 24, part 3, p. 2.

Whiting, David A. 1998. "Male Pattern Hair Loss: Current Understanding." *International Journal of Dermatology* 37: 561–66.

Whittington, Craig J., Tim Kendall, Peter Fonagy, et al. 2004. "Selective Serotonin Reuptake Inhibitors in Childhood Depression: Systematic Review of Published and Unpublished Data." *Lancet* 363: 1311–45.

WHO (World Health Organization). 1994. *International Classification of Diseases* (ICD-10). Geneva: WHO.

Wilcox, Sarah. 2001. "Scientific Communities, Gay Communities, and the Production of Knowledge: The Social Construction of Biological Ideas about Same-Sex Sexuality." Ph.D. diss., University of Pennsylvania.

Wilkes, Michael S., Robert A. Bell, and Richard L. Kravitz. 2000. "Direct-to-Consumer Prescription Drug Advertising: Trends, Impact, and Implications." *Health Affairs* 19 (2): 110–28.

Williams, Simon J. 2001. "Sociological Imperialism and the Profession of Medicine Revisited: Where Are We Now?" *Sociology of Health and Illness* 23 (2): 135–58.

——. 2002. "Sleep and Health: Sociological Reflections on the Dormant Society." *Health* 6 (2): 173–200.

——. 2005. *Sleep and Society: Sociology Ventures into the (Un)known.* London: Routledge.

Williams, Simon J., and Michael Calnan. 1996. "The 'Limits' of Medicalization: Modern Medicine and the Lay Populace in 'Late Modernity.'" *Social Science and Medicine* 42: 1609–20.

Wilson, Duff. 2005. "New Blood Pressure Guidelines Pay Off for Drug Companies." *Seattle Times.* Pp. 2–5 in special reprint of "Suddenly Sick," a series published June 26–30.

Wojnowski, Leszek. 2006. "Letter." *New England Journal of Medicine* 354: 2297.

Wolkenberg, Frank. 1987. "Out of a Darkness." *New York Times Magazine*, 11 October, 62, 66, 68–70, 82–83.

Wolpe, Paul R. 2002. "Treatment, Enhancement, and the Ethics of Neurotherapeutics." *Brain and Cognition* 50: 387–395.

Wolraich, Mark L., Scott Lindgren, et al. 1990. "Stimulant Medication Use by Primary Care Physicians in the Treatment of Attention Deficit Hyperactivity Disorder." *Pediatrics* 86: 95–101.

Wood, D. R., F. W. Reimherr, Paul H. Wender, and G. E. Johnson. 1976. "Diagnosis and Treatment of Minimal Brain Dysfunction in Adults." *Archives of General Psychiatry* 33: 1453–60.

Worcester, Nancy, and Marianne H. Whatley. 1992. "The Selling of HRT: Playing on the Fear Factor." *Feminist Review* 41 (summer): 1–26.

Writing Group for the Women's Health Initiative Investigators. 2002. "Risks and Benefits of Estrogen Plus Progestin in Healthy Postmenopausal Women: Principal Results from the Women's Health Initiative Randomized Controlled Trial." *Journal of the American Medical Association* 288: 321–33.

——. 2004. "Effects of Conjugated Equine Estrogen in Postmenopausal Women with Hysterectomy: The Women's Health Initiative Randomized Controlled Trial." *Journal of the American Medical Association* 291: 1701–12.

www.ahrp.org. "Alliance for Human Research Protection."

www.androgel.com.

www.chadd.org. "Children and Adults with Attention Deficit/Hyperactivity Disorder."

www.chadd.org/AM/Template.cfm?Section=Reports1&Template=/CM/ContentDisplay.cfm&
ContentID=1771. "2005 Annual Report."

www.consensus.nih.gov/1998/1998AttentionDeficitHyperactivityDisorder110html.htm. "Diagnosis
and Treatment of Attention Deficit Hyperactivity Disorder." NIH Consensus Development
Conference Statement, November 16–18, 1998.

www.FSD-Alert.org. "Female Sexual Dysfunction (FSD): A New Medical Myth."

www.GIDreform.org. "GID Reform Advocates."

www.help4adhd.org/faqs.cfm#faq4. "I'm an adult; doesn't AD/HD only affect children?"

www.hormoneshop.org.

www.mindfreedom.org. "United Action for Human Rights in Mental Health."

www.narth.com. "National Association for Research and Therapy of Homosexuality."

www.nccam.nih.gov. "National Center for Complementary and Alternative Medicine."

www.paxil.com.

www.p-d-r.com/ranking/WoodMac_Top100.pdf. "Top 100 Ethical Drugs by Sales."

www.pseudobulbar.com. "Pseudobulbar Affect Clinical Trials."

www.strattera.com/1_4_adult_adhd/1_4_adult.jsp. "Adult ADHD."

www.vital-solutions.com.

www.worldhealth.net. "American Academy of Anti-Aging Medicine."

Wyden, R. 1994. Testimony before the House Committee on Business, Subcommittee on Regulation, Business Opportunities, and Technology, on the Questionable Practices in Drug Industry
Marketing and Promotion, 12 October, 106th Cong., 1st sess.

Yalom, Marilyn. 1997. *A History of the Breast.* New York: Knopf.

Young, Alan. 1995. *The Harmony of Illusions: Inventing Post-Traumatic Stress Disorder.* Princeton:
Princeton University Press.

Zametkin, Alan J., and Monique Ernst. 1999. "Problems in the Management of Attention-Deficit-
Hyperactivity Disorder." *New England Journal of Medicine* 340: 40–46.

Zametkin, Alan J., Laura L. Liebenauer, G. A. Fitzgerald, A. C. King, et al. 1993. "Brain Metabolism in Teenagers with Attention-Deficit Hyperactivity Disorder." *Archives of General Psychiatry* 50: 333–40.

Zametkin, Alan J., Thomas E. Nordahl, Michael Gross, et al. 1990. "Cerebral Glucose Metabolism
in Adults with Hyperactivity of Childhood Onset." *New England Journal of Medicine* 323 (20):
1361–66.

Zimmerman, Susan. 1998. *Silicone Survivors: Women's Experiences with Breast Implants.* Philadelphia: Temple University Press.

Zito, Julie Magno, Daniel J. Safer, Susan dos Reis, et al. 2000. "Trends in the Prescribing of
Psychotropic Medications to Preschoolers." *Journal of the American Medical Association* 283:
1025–1030.

———. 2002. "Rising Prevalence of Antidepressants among US Youths." *Pediatrics* 109: 721–27.

———. 2003. "Psychotropic Practice Patterns for Youth: A Ten-Year Perspective." *Archives of Pediatric and Adolescent Medicine* 157: 17–25.

Zola, Irving Kenneth. 1972. "Medicine as an Institution of Social Control." Pp. 404–14 in Peter Conrad (ed.), *The Sociology of Health and Illness: Critical Perspectives,* 6th ed. New York: Worth.

————. 1991. "The Medicalization of Aging and Disability." Pp. 299–315 in *Advances in Medical Sociology*. Greenwich, CT: JAI.

Zorpette, Glenn. 2000. "All Doped Up—and Going for the Gold." *Scientific American*, May 20–22.

Zucker, Kenneth. 1990. "Gender Identity Disorders in Children: Clinical Descriptions and Natural History." Pp. 3–23 in Ray Blanchard and Betty Steiner (eds.), *Clinical Management of Gender Identity Disorders in Children and Adults*. Washington, D.C.: American Psychiatric Press.

Zucker, Kenneth, and Susan Bradley. 1995. *Gender Identity Disorder and Psychosexual Problems in Children and Adolescents*. New York: Guilford.

Zwillich, Todd. 2005. "CDC: Obesity Is Still an Epidemic." http//:www.webmd.com/content/Article/106/108330.htm.

Index

Page numbers in *italics* refer to tables.

About the Author

Peter Conrad is the Harry Coplan Professor of Social Sciences at Brandeis University. He received his Ph.D. in sociology from Boston University. He is the author or coauthor of more than a hundred journal articles and chapters as well as nine books, including *Deviance and Medicalization: From Badness to Sickness*; *Having Epilepsy: The Experience and Control of Illness*; *Sociology of Health and Illness: Critical Perspectives* (seven editions); and *The Double-Edged Helix: Social Implications of Genetics in a Diverse Society*. At Brandeis he was chair of the Department of Sociology for nine years and is currently chair of the interdisciplinary program "Health: Science, Society, and Policy." Professor Conrad received the 1981 Charles Horton Cooley Award from the Society for the Study of Symbolic Interaction for *Deviance and Medicalization* and the 2004 Leo G. Reeder Award from the American Sociological Association for "outstanding contributions to medical sociology."